Copyright 2019 by the author of this book Sean Hannon.

All rights reserved.
Published 2019.
Printed in the United States of America.

All rights reserved. No portion of this book may be reproduced, stored in a retrieval system, or transmitted in any form or by any means – electronic, mechanical, photocopy, recording, scanning, or other – except for brief quotations in critical reviews or articles, without the prior written permission of the author.

ISBN 978-1-950647-24-8

Publisher's Cataloging-in-Publication data

Names: Hannon, Sean, 1949, author.
Title: Don't take advice from fat doctors! : The Honesty Diet : shed the lies keeping us fat, sick, and in pain / Dr. Sean Hannon.
Description: First trade paperback original edition. | Parker [Colorado] : Bookcrafters, 2019.
Identifiers: ISBN 978-1-950647-24-8
Subjects: LCSH: Self-care, Health. | Pain—Diet therapy. | Weight loss—Popular works.
BISAC: HEALTH & FITNESS / Diet & Nutrition / Diets.
Classification: LCC RM216 | DDC 613.21—dc22

Illustrations by Greg Johnson.
Cartoon provided by CartoonStock.com.

Publishing assistance by BookCrafters,
Parker, Colorado
www.bookcrafters.net

Don't Take Advice From *Fat* Doctors!

Shed the Lies Keeping Us Fat, Sick, and in Pain

The Honesty Diet™

Dr. Sean Hannon

Medical Disclaimer

I am not your doctor! This book is intended to teach a philosophy about health – a belief system many health professionals may strongly disagree with.

This book does not constitute a doctor-patient relationship in any way, shape, or form. The author, publisher, and distributors specifically disclaim any liability allegedly incurred from the use or application of the contents of this book. Always consult your family doctor before beginning any new health practice or regime.

Acknowledgements

Drs. Joel Carmichael, Jason Markle, and Dan Murphy for their guidance in helping me get back on my feet.

Inspirational Acknowledgements

Over the years, I have found it fascinating that many comedians seem to have a far greater understanding about health than many health professionals. Indeed, these comedians have taught me much about health by humorously articulating the absurd logic many Americans embrace regarding the poor health and obesity epidemic of the United States. These comedians have provided me not only with much laughter and entertainment, but also with much of the inspiration behind this book. Among those I would like to thank include: Jay Leno, Bill Maher, Bill Burr, the late and great George Carlin, and many more.

I would also like to acknowledge the work of Stephen Covey and Anthony Robbins. Their works have been instrumental to me for over a quarter century. As such, they are cited and referenced with some frequency in this book.

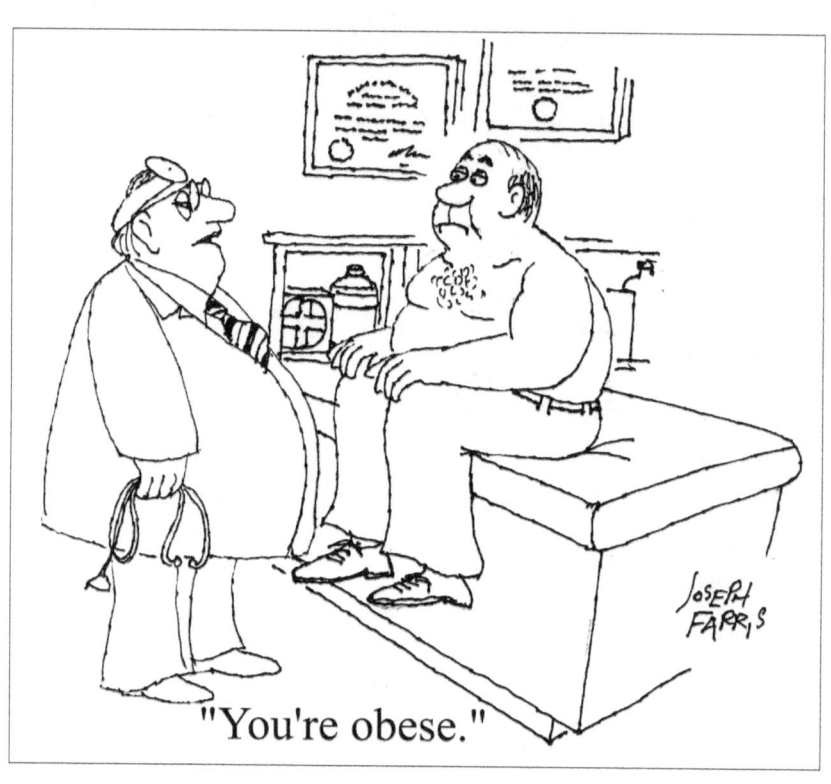

Contents

Author's Note..i
Introduction: A Word About "Science"......................iii

    Chapter 1   Meeting Pain...1

Section One: Reaching The Honesty Point™

    Chapter 2   A *Willingness* to Think Differently..........17
    Chapter 3   Reclaiming Our Capacity to *Think*..........28
    Chapter 4   Getting Results..38
    Chapter 5   Focus...46
    Chapter 6   Honesty..55
    Chapter 7   Awareness...72
    Chapter 8   Language Lies...93
    Chapter 9   Choice, Decision & Action.......................103
    Chapter 10 Values...122
    Chapter 11 It's What's on the *Outside* That Counts!..133
    Chapter 12 The *Big* Language Lie..............................138

Section Two: A New Perspective From The Honesty Point™

Chapter 13 The Honesty Point..................................163
Chapter 14 The Myth of Genetics............................169
Chapter 15 Being Fat Is a Choice..............................187
Chapter 16 Addiction Is a Choice.............................200
Chapter 17 Longevity Is a Choice.............................212
Chapter 18 Cancer is a Choice..................................229

Section Three: Practicing The Honesty Diet™

Chapter 19 Introduction to The Honesty Diet.........245
Chapter 20 Power, Control & Choices.....................256
Chapter 21 Belief Without Thought.........................270
Chapter 22 Priorities: The "Big Rocks" of Health...291
Chapter 23 Food Principles of The Honesty Diet...307
Chapter 24 Decide..347

Author's Note (2007)

This book frequently speaks in generalities. It does so for the sake of simplicity and clear communication. For example, I use the term "doctors" generically and mean for it to apply to all kinds of physicians including, but not limited to, chiropractic physicians, osteopathic physicians, medical physicians, and naturopathic physicians.

This book has three sections. Some might find Sections Two and Three easier to follow than Section One. However, Section One is critical to understanding and benefiting from The Honesty Diet. Though I have tried my very best, I concede that portions of Section One may be challenging at times. Just stick with it and it will pay off later. Take your time and read slowly. Don't skim. "Getting this" is really important to your health and well-being. Sections Two and Three will not mean as much to you if you haven't carefully embraced Section One.

Author's Note (2019)

I wrote *The Honesty Diet* in 2007. For a number of reasons, it was never published. After permitting some friends to read the draft some 12 years later, I was encouraged to reconsider putting it out for public consumption. Why? "Because it still holds up," they say. "In fact, it is more relevant than ever." I had wanted to write a book that would hold up over time. Apparently, I succeeded.

Everything I wrote 12 years ago was and still is accurate and I continue to stand behind its content today. Perhaps more importantly, nothing has changed. The problem has only gotten bigger – literally and figuratively. Americans are even fatter than they were 12 years ago. They have learned nothing and have made no progress. This book explains why this trend continues and tells you what you can do about it.

So, while there very much may be a *need* for this book, I am still uncertain there is a *desire* for this book. Nonetheless, here it is for your consideration. Take it or leave it. I don't care. It makes no difference to me at all. However, it very well could be the turning point you've been needing, and possibly seeking, in your life for a very long time.

I am no longer in practice and I'm not publishing this book with any intent of launching a career based on its content. I would just like it out there. Furthermore, I wish to make myself even more accountable to its contents and philosophy. I'm human and, therefore, fallible. I, too, can perpetually increase my own degree of honesty and improve my own health decisions.

Even though some people I have referenced or quoted have passed away since I wrote *The Honesty Diet*, and even though some statistics may have fluctuated somewhat since 2007, I have left that information unchanged for the 2019 publication purely for perspective purposes. This perspective only strengthens the main points of the book. Enjoy.

Dr. Sean Hannon, DC
September 2019

~ Introduction ~

A Word About "Science"

Many people read early draft versions of this book. Afterward, the most common suggestion I received was to add more scientific references to make the arguments I present more "credible." I firmly disagreed with these suggestions and refused to add more scientific references even though I have a strong background in research and it would have been very easy to have heeded their advice. From my point of view, adding more scientific references would, in fact, make the book *less* credible because "science" changes and contradicts itself each and every year with the advent of new and allegedly "better" studies.

Citing dozens and dozens of scientific references is what authors of almost every other health book do. And that hasn't really helped now, has it? We're still sick, fat, and in pain. I propose the answer to our health problems will not be found in more *science*, but in *honesty* and in *thinking*.

What we will explore in this book are principles within a *belief system* – not here today, gone tomorrow conflict-of-interest-ridden research studies and statistics. What we will discover is that true principles of health are a product of honesty and thinking.

Citing additional scientific references would in many ways defy the very purpose of this book. This book is meant to encourage people to think for themselves about their health and well-being. When you rely upon what lies internally, principles of health emerge. When you rely on the external – like the most recent scientific study, which, will likely be contradicted by a later study – you're just blowing with the prevailing wind of the day. This book's laurels do not rest upon any transient scientific information that will likely be found to be inaccurate within a year or so. Its underlying assumptions derive from honesty and thinking, not from windsock science.

~ 1 ~

MEETING PAIN

"What's the matter?" a friend said to me.

"I'm not sure. I've got a strange feeling in my low back. I don't think I'm going to be able to walk my dogs tomorrow," I replied.

"Crap. What did you do to it?"

"Nothing I'm aware of. It'll probably be okay in a day or so."

But it wasn't okay in a day or so. I had experienced many moderate episodes of low back trouble over the past several years and they had been increasing in frequency. This time it would last well over 365 days. And over the course of that year I would progress from moderate discomfort to difficulty walking and sitting, to no standing, sitting or walking at all, to excruciating, unbearable round-the-clock pain, to at one point not sleeping at all for almost five days straight. Over time I would progress to some limited walking with the heavy use of one of those "senior" walkers, to many months of relying on a cane and back brace, and finally back to walking, again, unassisted.

The most common questions I was asked were, "How did you injure your spine? Was it a car accident or a weight lifting injury?" I tried to explain that no singular event had torn my spinal discs. It was a progressive deterioration due to years and years of dishonesty and neglect. Then one day in early 2006, I came home from working out at the gym (without incident) and by the next day I could barely walk. The pain got worse and worse over the next several weeks until eventually I could no longer stand at all. This was incredibly embarrassing for me because I am a doctor, and rather ironically, a chiropractic physician. I had spent four years studying human physiology, particularly the health and mechanics of the spine. Yet, here I was, unable to walk. I felt like a complete phony. How could I ever practice again with such difficulty walking and in so much pain?

I had now taken up full-time residence atop my sturdy wooden coffee table in my living room and shared the room with my two dogs. I slept there for months. On that coffee table, I slept, ate, brushed my teeth, shaved, and tried to work on other sources of income I had been creating. The only thing I didn't do there was go to the bathroom – although I would have if I could have figured out a way to do so.

Absolutely no position I moved my body into was pain free. The least painful position was face down on the coffee table with my hips hanging off the long edge and my knees on the ground. I had nonstop, chronic, aching pain twenty-four hours a day, seven days a week for several months. There was no escaping the pain and I refused to take any drugs to treat the pain. When people asked why I wouldn't take any pain medication, I explained it was because while drugs may temporarily relieve pain, they actually slow down the healing process. Drugs also generate a false sense of security. Most people (including myself at times) erroneously assume that the absence of pain means the problem is gone, which leads many people to abuse drugs. They take the drug and when the pain goes away within 30 to 60 minutes they return to the activity causing the pain in the first place. I wanted to do anything and everything possible to heal this problem as fast as I could, and that meant no drugs.

My injury was quite serious. According to an MRI, one of the disc herniations was occluding about 80% of the spinal cord at one spinal level. As a result, I couldn't hold up my own body weight. Simple activities like going to the bathroom were a major challenge. Crawling across the floor, it would take me close to ten minutes to reach the bathroom — just fifteen feet away, all the while virtually screaming in pain. This occurred each and every time I needed to go to the bathroom. It wasn't really a true crawl to the bathroom. That hurt too much. It was more of a sliding on the floor a few inches at a time on my back or on my side. Of course, trying to stand up after finally reaching the bathroom was a feat in itself. A walker was placed in the bathroom next to the toilet so when I did eventually reach the bathroom, I had something sturdy to climb up.

The Honesty Diet

Once there, moving my bowels was almost impossible. I couldn't sit down at all because it hurt too much to sit. Bearing down was completely out of the question, and trying to get my pants back on afterward was incredibly difficult and often took over several minutes. When I did succeed, I then slid or crawled my way back to my makeshift home base, which was, of course, the coffee table. This process continued for several months with little noticeable progress.

When you can't walk for months at a time, you find yourself with a lot of time to think. There are only so many movies you can watch or books you can read before your mind starts to play tricks on you. One day, while I was by myself, the room was quiet, the TV was off (I now hated that thing), and the dogs, instead of being walked, were taking yet another afternoon nap. I was lying on my coffee table. Being depressed is tough for me because I am, in general, a happy person, but after two months of not being able to walk at all, I was reaching a breaking point. Suddenly I heard a voice say to me. *"Why do you think you're in the position you're in?"* My forehead creased. Did I just dream that? It's possible, I thought. I had been drifting in and out of consciousness, because sleep was so inconsistent. A few minutes later I heard the voice again. *"Why do you think you're in the position you're in?"* I looked around the room. There was no one else in the room. It was definitely a voice in my head, not my own voice but someone else's.

"What did you say?" I responded silently.

Just to be clear, I was very aware this was a conversation occurring purely in my head. There is no need to call the people with straitjackets. I heard the voice, again. *"I said, why do you think you're in the position you're in?"*

"Because I tore two of my spinal discs. Why else?"

"No," the voice stated sternly. *"That isn't the real answer. That isn't the whole truth, is it, Sean? Tearing your discs is only a description of what happened. My question to you was why. Why are you in the situation you are in?"*

"Who are you?" I asked, now wondering how insane this conversation would be if I were having it out loud.

"You know who I am. But, so that we don't waste any more time, why don't you just call me Pain."

"Pain? Your name is Pain?"

"No. Pain is not my real name. You're talking to yourself, so my real name is Sean. But, as you well know, you haven't been paying attention to me. I am the pain you've been experiencing. Considering we've been together nonstop, twenty-four hours a day for the past few months, I thought maybe we should eventually talk to each other."

"Talk to each other? You think I should talk to you… my pain?"

"Yes. I thought maybe if I separated myself from you for a while and we had a conversation together as separate entities you might see yourself and our shared predicament differently. Then maybe you'd learn something about this experience and actually fix it. So, now that we've gotten introductions out of the way, let's get back to the question at hand. Why are you in the situation you're in?"

"What did you mean when you said I'm not paying attention to you?"

"I can see this is going to take a while. You're not quite ready for absolute honesty yet, are you? Obviously, a part of you is

ready to make a change. Otherwise, I wouldn't be here and we wouldn't even be having this conversation. What I mean by 'you're not paying attention to me' is that you're not listening to what I'm trying to tell you. How long have I been talking to you?"

"How long have you been talking to me? For about two minutes."

"No. That's not what I mean. Yes, we've been talking to each other in English for about two minutes. But what I mean is, how long have you and I been communicating with each other?"

"About two or three months?"

"When you say it like that – as a question – then you already know that isn't the true answer, don't you?"

"I suppose."

"So how long have we really been communicating with each other?"

"A few years…"

"Just a few?"

"Okay. More than a few."

"How long exactly, Sean? Be honest."

"Since I was 17 years old."

"Bingo! Since you were seventeen. You first hurt your spine moving a heavy theater prop. That means we've been communicating with each other for many years. But, I'm the one who's been doing most of the talking. Overwhelmingly, you just ignore me. Do you remember when you were a teenager and your back hurt so much you couldn't get out of bed one morning or walk through the mall with your friends? You had to go lie down on a bench every twenty minutes."

"Yeah, I remember that."

Don't Take Advice From Fat Doctors!

"Do you remember not being able to walk for almost a week shortly after finishing your clinical internship?"

"Yes."

"Well, that was me, too. I was trying to talk to you then also. But you still wouldn't listen. You just kept pushing through me. No pain, no gain – isn't that your motto? You just kept thinking I would eventually go away. You were very stubborn. It has taken me this long to get you to talk to me. You were able to ignore me quite well, I'd say, through all those years and years of weight lifting, jogging, and martial arts. You had some pretty good years in there where we wouldn't talk with each other often, but I was always there, wasn't I?"

"Yep."

"So, are you ready to really talk yet?"

"OK, Pain," I said. "So what do you want to talk about? What are you doing here? Why are you talking to me now?"

"I'm here to help you. I've always been here to help. That's my purpose. That's my function. Most people treat me the same way you do. They think I'm just a nuisance, that I have no purpose. But that isn't true. You can't just ignore me year after year and think I'll eventually go away. The fact of the matter is, I'm here. I'm here now and speaking to you in plain English so we can more effectively communicate with each other. I'm going to help you get back on your feet. I'm going to help you heal completely. But first you need to start perceiving me as something to help you, not as something to be stifled. If we're going to do that I'm going to need you to do something you haven't done for a very long time."

"What's that?"

"I'm going to ask you to be honest."

The Honesty Diet

"Honest?"

"*Yes, honest. The reason why you can't sit, can't stand, can't walk and hurt so much is because you have been chronically dishonest about your back health for years. And, just because you're a doctor doesn't mean you get a 'get out of jail free' card. You have to follow the rules, too.*"

"OK. What do I need to do?"

"*First, you need to acknowledge out loud that the situation you're in is ENTIRELY your fault. Your spinal discs tore because you were being dishonest. The reason why you are in the position you are in is because you've been ignoring me. I've been trying to tell you for years by giving you pain... lots of it! But you kept ignoring me. Finally, when I couldn't stand being ignored anymore, I tore your discs. It seemed the only way I could get you to pay attention to me was to take almost everything else away from you.*"

"You had to take away my ability to stand and walk?"

"*I have your attention now, don't I? Honestly, would you ever have paid attention to me otherwise?*"

"Probably, not," I admitted. Pain was right. I'd always been a very go-go, nonstop kind of person for years. Every time I experienced this pain I'd just push through it. It never really occurred to me that there was something important Pain was trying to tell me. I always thought pain was an unimportant nuisance.

"*I don't mean to wreck your life at such a young age, but if I didn't immobilize you now, there's a good chance you would have been much worse later. But don't be too hard on yourself. You're actually much better off than most people. At least you were smart and refused to take drugs. Most people simply take drugs when they have pain. That's just like stuffing a sock in my mouth. I'm still there, they just can't hear me. Take drugs for too long and that is when people get themselves into real trouble. So are we going to do this, or what? Are you going to acknowledge your back pain as your fault?"*

"One of my colleagues suggested I may not have the genetics to regenerate some kinds of tissue fibers," I protested.

"That's bullshit, and you know it. If you continue to blame something or someone other than yourself, you're never going to heal."

"OK. You're right. This is my fault. I did this to myself."

"Out loud. Say it out loud," Pain insisted.

"Why do I have to do that?"

"Because saying something out loud is a sign of commitment and of honesty. Because, otherwise, this is only a conversation we are having inside your head. Saying it out loud will make it become more real."

"Okay, fine. This is my fault! I did this to myself! I've been ignoring my spinal health for years, and I have earned every bit of this pain and immobility! I chose this!"

"Well done," Pain said. *"Now, we can finally begin to heal."*

Over the next few months, I had many conversations like this with Pain. Pain continued to help me recognize that I had been ignoring my own spinal health for quite some time. I knew I had some spine damage from years ago. That is what led me to become a doctor in the first place. But I had come to realize I'd been putting everything else in my life ahead of my own health, particularly as it related to my spine. I was more focused on my career, growing businesses, investments, and hobbies than I was on my own health. As a result, it was my health that vanished.

I quickly learned how important my dialogue with Pain was and how valuable pain is with regard to health and healing. Over the next several months Pain and I started to develop an intimate partnership with each other. He helped me recognize all the things I had been doing for years that aggravated him, and he helped me recognize all the things I wasn't doing for myself that needed to be done if I was to one day return to sitting, standing, walking, and hopefully being a completely functional, athletic adult.

Pain made me acknowledge, write down, and say out loud all the lies I had been telling myself about my spinal health. Strangely, just this process of acknowledging these things seemed to propel me forward. Our partnership grew and became more and more acute. Pain agreed to give me immediate feedback on things I was doing in order to get better, and on things I needed to stop doing. For example, I still couldn't hold myself upright or walk without assistance, but at the same time, we knew I couldn't just lie around all day. I had to move my body in order to heal. The less I moved the more other parts of my body would continue to atrophy and that would just make me worse in the long run.

Pain introduced me to swimming. Pain explained that if I could get to the pool each day and just float around for an hour or so, my spine could get some relief and modest exercise without having to hold up my body weight. Within six months of going to the pool daily, I found I could swim over a mile in less than one hour, even though I still couldn't walk 100 yards.

As time passed, Pain and I developed such rapport with each other that Pain no longer had to speak English to me. We could almost read each other's thoughts. We were becoming one again. The separation between us was dissipating. Our dialogue became visceral and intuitive instead of verbal. Over time, we developed what we came to call a "visceral intelligence" – the ability to determine cause and effect in our body simply by learning to practice honesty and thinking.

Pain also helped me recognize that I needed more people on my team to help me heal. I was able to accelerate my healing by consulting with a talented medical physician on the East Coast by telephone. Through some sophisticated, proprietary blood analysis, she showed me why some elements in my blood were actually preventing my tissues from healing. We fixed the problem, not with drugs, but with nutrition. She agreed that drugs wouldn't address the real problem. But, by changing what I chose to put in my body, my body began to heal.

When I was strong enough, I began undergoing something called spinal decompression therapy, a non-surgical physiotherapy that rehydrates spinal discs over time. *"Is the reason why you are in your predicament because your spinal discs are dehydrated?"* Pain asked me.

"Yes," I replied.

"Good. Then, proceed."

Perhaps most importantly, Pain was extremely helpful in teaching me how to ignore bad health advice, especially that which came from well-intentioned but ignorant friends and family. One of the most common suggestions I got from these well-intentioned people was, "Why don't you go have surgery?" At times like these, Pain was the one who would whisper in my ear, "*Do you really believe the reason why you are in your predicament is because you haven't had enough surgery? Is that what the problem is? You have a surgery shortage?*"

"No. Of course, not," I would respond.

"*Then ignore these people. They don't know what they're talking about.*"

"But won't removing the spinal disc or part of it help get rid of the pain?"

"*Maybe. But do you think the spinal disc is there by accident, by mistake?*"

"No. It's supposed to be there."

"*Then how will removing it help heal your spine? How will removing your disc or part of it make it healthier and function properly?*"

"It won't."

"*Very good. That's the right answer. You're on the right path. You know what to do. Having surgery will not remove the behaviors and choices which brought you into this state of pain. Surgery would be cheating, and there's a good chance it'll lead to more problems and negative consequences later on. Just keep going. You're making tremendous progress because you're being honest with yourself.*"

I have come to appreciate the discomfort Pain brought me. I consider his messages an early warning system. If my spine begins to feel sore and achy, there must be a reason for it. It almost always means, "*Pay attention to me.*" I, like so many other people with different kinds of health challenges, was ignoring the message Pain was sending me. Only after Pain finally took away my ability to sit, walk, and stand and only after he spoke to me in English did I truly realize how valuable pain is.

This book is going to take you through a process Pain and I developed over the course of a whole year of healing. It is a process of self-honesty and self-exploration that can help you reach your health goals, whatever they may be.

Pain taught me how to heal myself with what we came to call The Honesty Diet. The Honesty Diet is not a science or a treatment. It is a *belief system* you create to produce rapid, unbelievable change in your life, whether that change is a journey of healing from an injury (as in my case), addressing a disease of some kind, or the chronic condition affecting most Americans today: obesity.

The lessons I learned can be applied to any health endeavor. And, since most people don't ever find themselves in a situation like mine, I have spent the majority of this book applying The Honesty Diet in a weight loss context. Since 66% of Americans are overweight, I thought this to be the most appropriate use of the principles of The Honesty Diet. But just remember, The Honesty Diet holds true for any health challenge.

I was told by many that if I didn't have surgery, I may never walk again. I was told I would never heal without taking drugs. I was told it was unlikely I could ever heal my spine and return to normal activities. *They were all wrong.* By following The Honesty Diet I achieved what everyone else said couldn't be done and have overwhelmingly returned to normal activities.

Everyone has a Pain inside of them; and the pain Pain

brings isn't necessarily just physical pain. In my case, Pain also came with tremendous emotional pain in the form of loss of control and self-esteem, and feelings of helplessness, weakness, and fragility. Whether your health challenge is chronic pain, a disease, or obesity, the principles of The Honesty Diet will apply to its resolution. You will learn while reading The Honesty Diet that we all have the power, the control, and the resources to solve our health challenges if we choose to recognize this power. Let's begin.

~ Section One ~

First Steps Toward The Honesty Point™

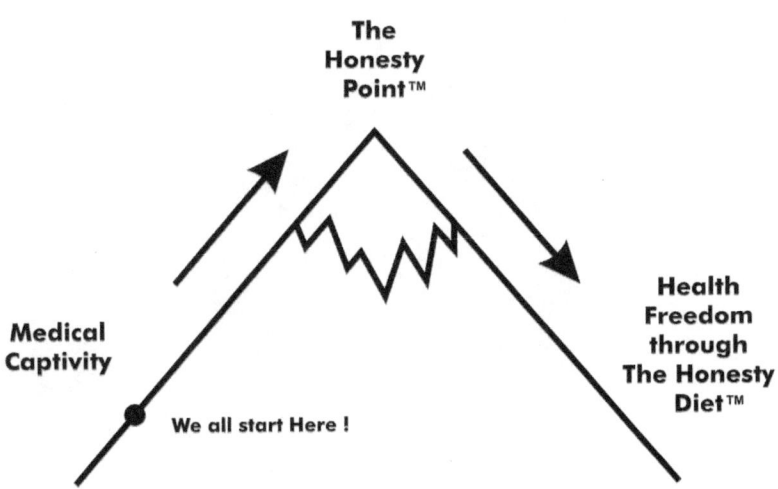

~ 2 ~

A WILLINGNESS TO THINK DIFFERENTLY

> *"The significant problems we face cannot be solved at the same level of thinking we were at when we created them."*
> - Albert Einstein

Albert Einstein said so many wonderful things throughout his life. Though he is largely remembered for his contributions to theoretical physics, I remember him most for his poignant, philosophical epigrams. The one above is my favorite. It appears frequently in many books and is meant to be thought provoking. However, far too often, authors place this quote somewhere in their book, but then rarely interpret or explore its meaning, relevance, and how it relates to the assertions in their book. Unfortunately, the reader often misses its significance.

The Honesty Diet

This quote has been instrumental to many successes in my life, once I really grasped its meaning. After I understood Einstein's meaning, many challenges and difficulties seemed to vanish overnight. Two other quotes express the same idea:

> *"Insanity: doing the same thing over and over again, and expecting a different result."*
> - Albert Einstein

> *"If you think the problem is outside of yourself, that, in and of itself, is the real problem."*
> - Stephen Covey

To me, all three of these quotes express the same life lesson: If you want to solve a problem, change something, or achieve a different result in any area of life, you must mentally *perceive the problem differently* from how you've perceived it in the past. You must recognize you have different *choices* regarding the dilemma, and therefore, you must make different *decisions* and take different *action* than you have in the past. But most importantly, you must *think* differently. What Einstein, Covey, and many others have repeatedly expressed is that: The way we *see* the problem is the problem. If we cannot *perceive* the problem differently from how we have in the past, we will *never* get a better result. The same holds true for our health. If we wish to tackle our health problems of today, we must first change the way in which we fundamentally "see" the problem. That can, at times, be a very uncomfortable process.

Each year, dozens of new books are published claiming to offer a new diet guaranteed to help people lose weight. And, each year many of the same people who bought last year's diet books also buy this year's diet books in high hopes of becoming healthy and losing weight they failed to lose last year. They keep doing the same thing over and over again – following diets and failing – yet they keep expecting a different result. If you want to get a different result, you must do things *differently* than you have in the past. More importantly, you must *think* differently than you have in the past. The Honesty Diet provides the means, the philosophy, and the mental distinctions to help us think *differently* about health and fitness.

Most new diet books basically revise or contradict previous diet books. Almost all of them communicate the idea that the reason why someone is unhealthy or overweight is because they aren't following the "right" diet – and, of course, what they mean by the "right" diet is whichever one they are currently peddling.

If you've tried diet after diet and continue to fail or have less than satisfactory results, perhaps you need to step outside your mental box, *think* differently, and ask yourself, "If these kinds of diets haven't helped me in the past, why would they help me now?" Maybe the reason every diet fails is not because of the *kind* of diet it is, but because of the *concept* of a diet – the idea that you are trying to lose weight and become healthy by means of a traditional diet in the first place!

After literally hundreds of diets have been offered to Americans over the past several decades, what do we have to show for it? The only *honest* answer is *more* fat Americans! That doesn't sound very successful to me. The problem isn't any given diet. The problem is a lack of *thinking* and the lack of courage to be *honest* with yourself about the real origins of health and fitness.

Most health books focus on the diet portion of their program. I believe that's why so many people fail to reach their goals while dieting. Losing weight and becoming healthy is first and foremost a *psychological* phenomenon, not a *physical* phenomenon. This is what most people simply do not understand. People gain weight and become sick largely because of how they think and feel about themselves. They have poor beliefs about health, how to achieve health, the amount of control they have in their lives, etc. To become healthy and to permanently lose weight, one's psychology must be addressed first.

There are countless books on what to *do* in order to be healthier. Eat this. Don't eat that. Take this drug. Take this herb. But this book is different. This book will *not* focus on what to *do*, but rather *how to think* about health. Not *what* to think, but *how* to think. This book is not going to tell you what foods to eat, which supplements to take, or what exercises to do. That is what virtually every other health book on the market touts, and – look around – it hasn't really worked now, has it? It hasn't worked because contrary to what most people believe, it is not the "doing" of these kinds of things that create health. Instead, this book will teach you how to answer questions yourself, like "What to eat?" Deep down, if you are being *honest*, thinking and paying attention, I contend you already know the answer. This book will show you how to do these three things: be honest, think, and pay attention so you can uncover those answers for yourself.

Our goal is not to all look like ripped, bodybuilders. That is something very different – a different kind of extreme from the one most of us are struggling with today. Rather, our goal is to get back to reasonable, healthy body proportions. To get back to the way average people looked in, say, the 1970s. Those were appropriate human body proportions.

Through a desperately needed rediscovery of *honesty*, this book can help plainly identify those things which prevent people from being healthy and then suggest how to overcome them. This book teaches how to ask yourself honest questions that produce honest answers – answers that can produce immediate change. These answers permit us to create health on our own, instead of relinquishing responsibility solely to those wearing white coats and stethoscopes.

This book, quite literally, is about how to *think* about health in order to *create* health. It is true, if people could simply learn to be honest and *think* about health, most of their health problems would vanish. For some time now we as a society have been conditioned *not* to think about health. It is a system that leads us to believe that we are at the mercy of the doctor-pharmaceutical industry and are destined to suffer within it.

Many people often think I'm joking when I suggest

few people really want to be healthy – that Americans are sick and fat simply because they *choose* to be. But, I assure them I am quite serious. Most people *value* things like career and entertainment more than they do their health, and that is exactly why so many are so sick and fat. Some readers may feel hurt or even offended by some of the non-politically correct statements you'll read in this book. However, if you feel offended by something you read, then you have a choice to make. You can either decide I'm a jerk, put down the book, and continue living the way you are, or you can *choose* to decide it's really a good thing you feel offended, because pain is almost always the impetus to all change.

Change is almost always uncomfortable. In fact, in many respects, comfort is the very opposite of change. So, if you say you want change, but at the same time you aren't willing to become uncomfortable in the process, then truth be told, you don't *really* want to change. When people come to me looking for help, I often see it as my job to help them reach a point of upset – a point we will come to call The Honesty Point.

The Honesty Point represents a specific mental state. A point at which one often experiences a revelation of sorts – an awareness, if you will – that through an acknowledgement of honesty, suddenly catapults one directly toward the health goals they seek but have struggled to achieve. Sometimes that goal is achieving substantial weight loss, sometimes it is getting out of chronic pain, and other times it means healing from disease. Things that once seemed impossible or unattainable suddenly begin to manifest with ease.

If someone is *fortunate* enough to become upset and disturbed – to reach The Honesty Point – then they have reached a point of opportunity, an opportunity to grow and to change. Unless one reaches The Honesty Point, one isn't likely to ever change. Becoming upset is often a sign of growth and a sign of progress. Like lifting weights – it kind of hurts, but it produces tremendous results. If you are not getting upset or uncomfortable, most likely no growth is taking place.

Reaching The Honesty Point is an enormous psychological achievement and it opens doors for tremendous change. Indeed, once reached, everything else becomes much, much easier. But it is often difficult to recognize this truth until that point is reached, and that is why so many people turn back in failure. They quit long before they reach The Honesty Point. Through each chapter we will come upon various, often challenging, awarenesses I suggest are required in order to become healthy. This book will show you how to quickly reach The Honesty Point so you can create for yourself the level of health and vitality you desire for you and your family. It isn't necessarily easy, but is well worth it.

Some may read this book and conclude there is nothing new in it. That it is all common sense. I firmly disagree. It's *good* sense, but it isn't *common* sense. Look around. Over two-thirds of Americans are fat, suffer from hypertension, and nearly that many are taking several drugs. It is currently estimated that one out of two people will develop heart disease, and one out of three people will develop cancer. Therefore, this book may contain simple, good sense, but it certainly isn't common!

Lastly, although I will try, I can't completely sell you on the ideas in this book just through the written word. Much of what I write about *must* be experienced, not just read about. So many people defensively claim they must be intellectually convinced about something and be guaranteed a successful outcome before they will take any action whatsoever. But so many things in life are rooted in experience and escape the written word. For example, try to describe a new color – not a different shade or combination of any existing colors, but an actual new color – a never seen before color. Tough, isn't it? In fact, it can't be done. It is impossible to conceive, much less describe a new color unless you first experience it. So, too, it is with the principles and beliefs found in this book. It may take you quite a while to reach The Honesty Point. However, eventually you will have to make a decision to either give this belief system a try, or not.

As such, it is important you not just read this book. You must actually do it. By simply *reading* you'll only acquire more mental knowledge. You may already have a great deal of mental knowledge, but still struggle with your weight or your health. More mental knowledge won't benefit you all that much unless you apply it as *visceral* knowledge or *visceral* intelligence. Visceral intelligence is a product of *experience*. Experience produces results, passive reading does not. Visceral intelligence is the ability to intuitively and accurately identify cause and effect in your body. Visceral intelligence is a product of *honesty* – and honesty *creates* health. Being fit and healthy and staying fit and healthy requires *visceral* intelligence and acting upon the belief system presented in this book.

Everyone has a strong, innate visceral intelligence, but for most it has been suppressed and buried by what we will learn to call *medical captivity*.

A Word About "Yeah, buts..."

You will draw greater benefit out of this book if you read it with a *willingness* to think differently, a *willingness* to become uncomfortable, and a *willingness* to explore new ideas. This book will likely challenge many of your current beliefs about health. So, don't talk your way out of the lessons of this book simply by trying to find fault with, or an exception to, a new and possibly uncomfortable awareness contained within it.

So many people read books and articles from an intellectual perspective of trying to find something wrong with what they are reading instead of trying to learn something new. It is almost as if they want to read something that says exactly what they already know! How does that help anyone?

Should you find yourself at some point saying things like, "*Yeah, but* that isn't always true" or "*Yeah, but* there is an exception to that," you might as well put down this book and spend your valuable time doing something else. People who are full of "Yeah, buts" aren't really trying to learn anything new or produce change. And, ironically, people who are full of "Yeah, buts..." often have big "butts," too.

The "Yeah, buts" of the world aren't interested in changing, but rather they use "Yeah, buts" to intellectualize their *existing* belief systems so they can talk themselves out of having to change. If you don't *want* to change, then don't! It makes no difference to me. But if you do want to change and improve your health from wherever it is now, you have to possess the *willingness* to explore new ways of looking at things, new ways of thinking of things, and new ways of taking action. Otherwise you'll just get the same results you've always been getting. And, that isn't why you are reading this book, is it?

Now *obviously*, exceptions can always be found. The trick, however, is to recognize when you are truly identifying an exception, and when you are just using "Yeah, buts…" as an excuse for not being *willing* to change or to think differently.

You can use the "Yeah, but" response as a litmus test. If you find yourself saying, "Yeah, but…" at any point, stop, take a deep breath, relax, and then get honest with yourself. Ask, "Why am I resisting this new idea? What *belief* do I currently have that is conflicting with what I am reading? What is it about this new idea that makes me uncomfortable?" Or, "What benefits do I get from *not* wanting to change?" Asking questions like these will help you get more out of reading this book when you find yourself resisting or outright rejecting some of its viewpoints.

You might also find some of your answers illuminating. "Yeah, buts" represent a point of resistance. A point of resistance is an opportunity for growth. Just like exercising a muscle, the last repetition, the most difficult repetition, is when growth initiates. When you start to hear the "Yeah, buts" in your head (and, I promise, you will), recognize that point of resistance as your opportunity – your point of growth. It is this "Yeah, but" phenomenon that often prevents people from reaching The Honesty Point. One cannot benefit from The Honesty Diet unless they first reach The Honesty Point.

~ 3 ~

RECLAIMING OUR CAPACITY TO THINK ABOUT HEALTH

Your Only Asset

Reclaiming our capacity to *think* about health is the first step of our journey to The Honesty Point. What is the one single thing you will have with you for your entire life no matter how long you live? Give up? It's your body. Your body is the one and only thing you will have for your *entire* life – from start to finish. Friends, spouses, family, careers, money, homes, and cars will all come and go. They are all transient things. Throughout the course of your life, even intangible things like feelings, thoughts, and beliefs will greatly change, and will come and go. Only your body will be with you the whole time.

Quite literally then, your body is the *only* asset you have. It is the vehicle which will transport you through life. However, you can't trade in this vehicle every few years for a new one. The one you have is the one you get. That's it. In which case, don't you think it would be a good idea to have a working knowledge of how to take care of your one and only asset?

Human physiology should be the most important subject taught in primary education K through 12. I would argue that understanding human physiology is even *more* important than reading, writing, and arithmetic. Think about it. How important are these three subjects if you're dead?

Growing up, most of us were taught that it is a doctor's responsibility to take care of our bodies. As a result, most of us have literally *outsourced* the maintenance of our bodies to the medical and pharmaceutical industries. This relinquishment is the *cause* of the problem. I have chosen not to participate in this outsourcing – this relinquishing of control – of my health. As a result I have not needed prescription medications, antibiotics, or vaccines for nearly 20 years now. That is not to say I wouldn't consider using these kinds of things if I determined there was an urgent need. But because of the daily decisions I make about basic health requirements: nutrition, exercise, sleep, and stress reduction; I haven't had any urgent need for medication in decades.

Learn about your body and it will benefit you. Learn about how your body works and it will serve you well. Choose not to learn about your body and you will harm and shorten your life. The best way to learn about how your body works isn't necessarily by becoming a doctor, but by being honest and becoming educated. After all, I know lots of doctors who are fat, unhealthy, and truly don't understand how the body works. They may

The Honesty Diet

understand how to follow flow charts and prescribe certain treatments based upon certain symptoms, but many lack a fundamental understanding of how the body works and heals. Not surprisingly, these same doctors are often not very healthy themselves. So why should we take advice from them?

It is also important to recognize that no one will care about you more than you will. You must take a vested interest in your health. You simply can't spend your life relying on doctors to maintain your health and still expect to stay healthy. Think about it. If medicine made us healthy, wouldn't it stand to reason that the people who take the *most* medicine should be the *healthiest* people? Is that the case? Think about people you know who take lots of medications. Are they the *healthiest* people you know, or the *sickest*? If your experience is anything like mine, then the people you know who take the most medications are usually the sickest people you know. Does that *really* make sense to you? Isn't medicine supposed to make people healthy?

When do you most often go to see a doctor? You either go when you are already sick (in which case you've already lost your health), or you go for the early detection of cancerous conditions. You may recognize these latter kinds of doctor visits by the more commonly used terms "wellness" visits and "preventive" checkups. Mind you, there is nothing "preventive" about cancer screenings. They don't *prevent* anything. They just tell you you might not have cancer... right now. Similarly, there is nothing "well" about wellness visits. All they can tell you is they can't find any diseases... yet.

These kinds of awarenesses will become increasingly obvious to you as we approach, reach, and pass The Honesty Point. It will be a journey well worth the time and *emotional* investment you make in this book. You will be pleasantly shocked by the freedoms, the choices, the empowerment, and the physical health benefits that will emerge as you release yourself from dishonest, auto-programmed beliefs preventing you from experiencing the levels of health you deserve.

The Naked Honest Truth

Real health begins by being honest. Dishonesty *creates* poor health. In order to be or become healthy we must learn to be honest with ourselves. When we are honest with ourselves about our current state of health, then and only then can we begin to improve our health. Like many addiction treatment programs state, "Nothing gets better until you admit you have a problem." So having said this, please do the following exercise with me:

I'm going to ask you to do something you may consider a little strange, perhaps even a bit uncomfortable. Remember: becoming uncomfortable is a sign of growth and opportunity. You don't have to do it right this minute; you can do it later if you'd like, but the sooner you do it the better. Go to a room with a full-length mirror, tightly close the blinds or curtains, and turn as many lights <u>on</u> as possible. Now, completely remove your clothes and stand in front of that full-length mirror. Yes, you have to open your eyes when you do this! Take a look. Take a good, long look. The mirror doesn't lie. For several

The Honesty Diet

minutes assess what is in front of you. Relax and really take the time to observe what you see. Then as objectively as you can, make note of what you see.

Do you like what you see? Does the image make you feel proud? Do you feel sexy? Do you think others would find you sexy? How does your skin look? How do your eyes look? Are they vibrant or tired looking? Do your eyes have bags under them? Do you look older than you really are? Would you say you look healthy? Are you fit? And, what I mean by fit is: Are you as fit as you'd like to be? Do you have much muscle tone? How is your posture? Now try this: look down. Can you see your feet without leaning over, or is there a large dome of flesh in the way? Can you see your abdominal muscles? Are you fat? Do you think others would say you're fat? If you have hair on your head, does it look healthy? Are you prematurely gray?

How is your skin tone and color? Do you see any scars or stretch marks from pregnancy or a caesarian scar from childbirth? Do you have any other scars from an injury or surgery? Do you have any tattoos or piercings other than your ears, perhaps? Just take a good look at yourself – really take it all in and evaluate. Contrary to what many of you were taught growing up, it is okay to judge yourself. *Honestly*, do you like what you see, overall? How does your image make you feel?

Now, don't put your clothes back on just yet. We're not quite finished. Here is the point of this exercise. What you see in the mirror is, quite literally, a reflection of your *health* – not your *fitness* (although that, too, is reflected in the mirror). More specifically, what you see there, naked, staring back at you is nothing more than the cumulative product of all of the choices you have made on a daily basis for weeks, months, years, maybe even decades – nothing more, nothing less. If you're really being *honest* with yourself, you also already know this to be true. *You are as fit and as healthy as you are currently committed to being.* Unless you have scars from something that happened to you or a deformity from birth, what you see in the mirror is, indeed, the product of *your* choices and decisions.

OK, I can already hear some of your objections. "That's not fair! There is nothing I can do about my height!" Or, "That is ridiculous! It's not my fault my eyes are brown!" Or, perhaps some of you are saying, "I can't help it if I have my father's ears." These are not the kinds of things I'm talking about. When I do this exercise myself (which I have, several times) I, too, say things like "I wish I were six-foot-two." I'm talking about those *other* things. I'm talking about things like muscle tone, skin quality, bags under the eyes, and body fat. You know, those things we all have control over, but sometimes *pretend* we don't or just *choose* to ignore?

Some of you might be objecting to this exercise for different reasons. Perhaps some are thinking, "What, do you expect me to look like, a movie star or something?" Or, "I look this way because I chose to have children." Others might be saying, "I look this way because I don't have time to exercise." Or, "I have to get up at 5 a.m. and I don't get home until 9 p.m.!" This is not being honest. Time, for example, is perhaps the only thing truly equal among all people on this planet. Excuses like these are not honest. It doesn't make any difference how wealthy you are, how busy you are, or what country you come from. All human beings have 24 hours each day. If you believe, for example, you don't have time to exercise, there is one, and only one, reason for it... you don't *value* exercise. If exercise were important to you, you would do it. It's that simple. Is this really an unfair statement on my part? I don't think so. The person who gets up at 5 a.m. and doesn't get home until 9 p.m. chose that job, that business, or that career. If the consequence of such a choice is there's no time to exercise, he or she may want to reevaluate their career decision. No "Yeah, buts..." please. Things are what they are. That person *chose* that situation, they can *choose* their way into a new and better situation.

After you have finished examining yourself in the mirror, what do you think? Did you like what you saw? I imagine some of you did, and some of you, maybe even most of you, did not. Maybe some of you are smiling and giving yourself a pat on the back. If so, great! If you are being really honest with yourself and you liked what you saw, congratulations! I hope you're proud, and you should be. You are already on your way. How about the rest of you? How do you feel, right now? Not so good? Terrible? Devastated, even? Well, now what? Where do you go from here? Don't worry, you just have to retrain yourself to be honest, and then reclaim your capacity to think about your health.

Medical Captivity

Learning to think about health is not difficult, but it often requires some initial instruction to help get back into the *habit* of thinking. We have, for so long, relinquished control of our health to the men and women in white coats that, in many respects, we have literally *forgotten* how to *think* about health. A similar phenomenon occurs when an animal raised in captivity has a difficult time surviving once released back into the wild. Much like these animals, we too have been raised in captivity – *medical* captivity.

Medical captivity has robbed us of our ability to *think* about health. Through a century-long, industry-coordinated marketing effort, we have been conditioned to believe we couldn't possibly know as much about health as a doctor does, and therefore we have no business addressing our health issues without first consulting a doctor.

We have been conditioned to believe that illness is an inconvenience needing to be swept away as soon as possible, so we can get back to doing what it was we were doing before we became sick. This is a *dishonest* and *naïve* way of looking at illness. Symptoms are the *language* of the body – a language with meaning and intent. Symptoms are the body's attempt to directly and loudly communicate with you. Therefore, we should listen to the voice of these symptoms, not just suppress them or ignore them.

We are constantly stifling the body's important messages. When we are tired, instead of resting, most of us drink coffee.

When we have diarrhea, instead of allowing the body to naturally rid itself of the culprit, we take an antidiarrhetic. When we are constipated, instead of hydrating our bodies, we take a laxative. When we have a cough or cold, instead of letting our bodies eject the bacteria or virus, we take cough suppressants and nasal decongestants. And, of course, when we are overweight, instead of losing weight we buy bigger clothes. It goes on and on.

Every time the body tries to tell us something important, most of us tell it to shut up and get back to work. This isn't very honest and, in fact, is the source of much illness and poor health. This dishonesty stems from a *belief* that sickness is primarily something that happens to us, instead of something we *voluntarily* develop through our daily choices.

Caroline Myss, Ph.D., author of *The Anatomy of Spirit*, once said something to the effect, "Illness and disease are the only socially acceptable forms of Western meditation." What I think she means is that far too often the only way people will ever look inward is *after* an illness has occurred. It never occurs to them that inward reflection, or what I call *inward honesty,* might actually help *prevent* the illness in the first place.

People who tend to think dealing with their health is a hassle are living life at a low level of health consciousness. I often ask these people, "*If you don't take care of your body, where in the world are you going to live?*" You'd be amazed at how many people actually don't understand this question. They often look at me like I've got six heads. They seem to forget that in order to live they need a healthy, functioning body.

Don't Take Advice From Fat Doctors!

We all have an inborn aptitude for *thinking* about health. It's just that for most of us, this innate ability has atrophied through generations of conditioned medical captivity. But for some of us, it hasn't. Even as a teenager, long before I became a doctor, I would see my mother taking drugs for headaches and would ask her, "Mom, do you think the reason why you have a headache is because there aren't enough drugs in your body? Does that really make sense to you?"

> *"How fortunate for leaders that men do not think."*
>
> – Adolf Hitler

In many respects, this quote could be restated today, "How fortunate for *doctors* that *patients* do not think." Medical captivity gives doctors a kind of job security. Past Surgeons General and many other experts have acknowledged if people would just take care of themselves as much as 70% of health problems, *including* cancer and heart disease, could be avoided altogether. It stands to reason that if people would just reclaim their ability to be honest and *think* about health, there would be little need for a doctor's services other than for emergency medical care.

~ 4 ~

GETTING RESULTS

Doers vs. Thinkers

Honesty and awareness must precede any actions taken toward health. Most people fail to achieve good health because they spend all their time "doing" instead of "thinking." They spend their health efforts avoiding carbohydrates, counting calories, taking supplements, or working out at the gym instead of preparing their mind and their thoughts for good health. Most fail to acknowledge, or were never taught, that *the healthy mental state is one of honest awareness,* and is the *prerequisite* for real, long-term health. Yet, few people condition themselves in this way to achieve good health. They fail to produce good health in their lives, because they simply do not understand how to make things happen or how to get successful results.

People who are successful in health, business,

relationships, or whatever have on some level mastered the ability to get results. Of course, they might not consciously realize their mastery, and it may not easily spill over from one area of life to the next.

The formula for good health is really quite simple, yet escapes most people's awareness. Good health is simply a function of mastering three simple, sequential steps. Skip any one of these steps and the desired result will not occur. Let's go over the process as a whole first. Then we can break each step down into its individual components.

Thought ➤ Decision ➤ Result

The formula progresses quite simply. *Thought* is the first *required* step. The *quality* of thought determines the *quality* of the second step – decision. The *right* thoughts will produce the *right* decisions, just as the *wrong* thoughts will produce the *wrong* decisions. Similarly, healthy thoughts will produce healthy decisions, and sick thoughts will produce sick decisions. *Decision*, and only decision, can produce *results*. Just as with thought, the *right* decision will produce the *right* results, and the *wrong* decision will produce the *wrong* results. In order to make the right decision, you must first have the right thoughts. So, in effect, it is the right thoughts that ultimately produce the right results, but only *through* the right decisions. Merely having the right thoughts cannot, in and of themselves, produce the right results.

The Honesty Diet

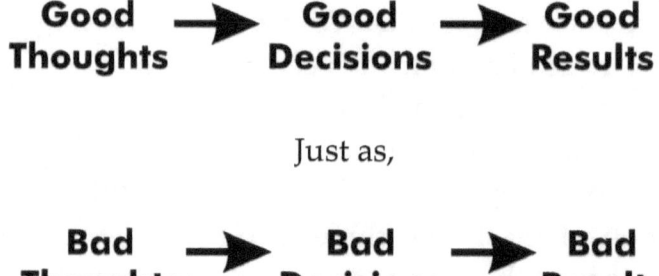

For example, many people believe smoking causes sickness. I disagree. Smoking is an action, an action that was the result of a sick decision. Therefore, the person was actually sick *before* they started smoking. The sick *thought* to start smoking is the real cause of the person's illness. The person was already sick. The sick thought produced the sick decision to smoke, which, in turn, produced the sick result (e.g. emphysema).

There are no shortcuts in getting successful results. Yet, that doesn't stop people from trying to take them. The most common shortcut looks like this:

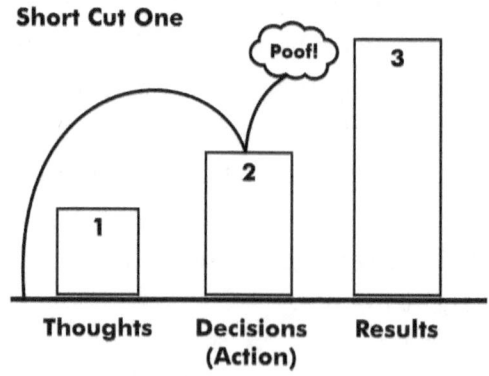

In this shortcut, people with good intentions try to skip the first step. That is, they try to achieve results by "doing" without first generating the necessary thoughts to produce the right decisions. Because they have skipped the first step, they usually burn out and are disappointed with their results. They "do," that is, they take lots of "action," however their efforts are usually poorly leveraged and without direction.

In trying to improve health, it might take the form of their doing numerous random exercises several times a week. But emotionally they really hate and resent doing those exercises. It could also be their exercise is unmeasured, done with poor form, or without control. They may eat the right foods, but they eat them from a perspective of *discipline* – a perspective from which they think they will become healthy by punishing themselves. This almost never works. Not only do they not enjoy the foods they select, but also they resent the reason why they're eating them.

It is no wonder these hard "doers" fail so often. They skipped the first step – thought. Even though they're working hard "doing," they're quite literally, *cheating* without being aware they are cheating.

Individuals who choose this road usually have similar physical attributes. They are more often, but not always, male, loud, aggressive, and "go-getters." I call them "hard-wired" people. They tend to believe the way to get ahead is through sheer physical force. Their motto is, "No pain, no gain." I used to be a proud, card-carrying member of this group.

The Honesty Diet

The other, less common, but perhaps more detrimental, shortcut looks like this:

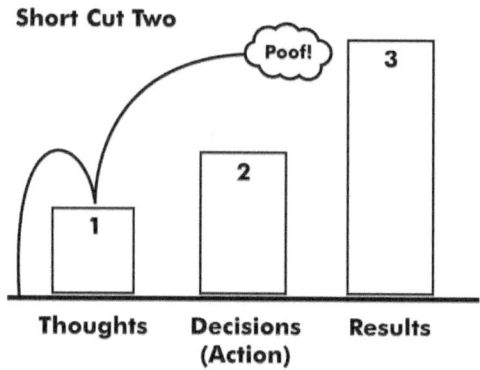

These people, also very well intentioned, definitely understand and value the importance of thought – the first step. To their credit, they fully embrace the importance of thought, and understand intellectually how *right* thoughts lead to the *right* results. However, they are very much the opposite of the "hard-wired" people. You could fairly easily and accurately refer to them as "soft-wired" people, or just "softies." These individuals tend to embrace spirituality, (though not necessarily religion) and tend to use words and phrases associated with spirituality. Frequently, they will make reference to "energies" and "universal forces." Often, they believe that *only* thought is required in order to manifest. They also tend to avoid physical effort. In general, softies don't like to sweat and tend to consider anything that might make them a bit uncomfortable, a form of punishment. More often than not, they are female, gentle, quiet, and frequently, very plump.

Softies have a tendency to ignore the missing ingredient toward their success. Softies are quite certain that if only their thoughts are good enough, then they can achieve their desires. The following is a true story, I think, will accurately illustrate the thinking pattern of a soft-wired person.

One evening, while attending an informal philosophical lecture in graduate school, one of my instructors, a wonderfully-talented, yet overweight doctor, attempted to argue that we all can accomplish any *physical* feat if only we could "vibrate" at a high enough "spiritual" level. When ask what she meant by this, she offered the following example:

"If I were to *raise my energy*, to truly *vibrate* at a *high enough level*," she said, "I could, instantaneously, create a thin body for myself."

"That's ridiculous," I objected. "If that were true, then why don't you do it right now?"

"Because I haven't reached that level of spirituality yet," she answered.

Try an exercise bicycle, I thought to myself. I was thoroughly disappointed in this instructor. Softies have a tendency to think "spiritual" means nonphysical. I have come to realize this is, often, nonsense. In fact, *physical* experience is, in many ways, the *essence* of spirituality. Softies, however, often refuse to recognize this, and that is why so many of them struggle physically.

For example, in the mid 1990s I went to hear a well-known author speak on the subject of spirituality at a

The Honesty Diet

convention I attended in New York City. A rather stout woman in the audience raised her hand and asked him, "What can I do to be more *spiritual*?"

His response was, "Take a walk in the sunshine."

"I know," she said, "but what I mean is, how can I attain a more spiritual existence?"

The speaker answered her again, "Eat an apple." The woman frowned. I guess she was looking for an answer like sit cross-legged, close your eyes and say "ohhhmmmm." She didn't understand the lesson this gentleman was sharing. The speaker, a former champion athlete, understood spirituality is just as much a physical experience as it is a nonphysical experience. Yet so many softies don't want to hear that, because they typically don't like physical exertion. That may be why so many of them are overweight.

So what this audience member and my former instructor don't seem to value is the second step in the manifesting: Decision! Decision is the *bridge* between the right thought and the right result. The only way to "vibrate" at a level high enough to lose weight is to *decide* and take *physical* action. My internal scoff, *try an exercise bicycle*, was, in fact, a fair and accurate suggestion. My instructor kept using the word "vibrate" as a nonphysical, spiritual term, when really the word "vibration" is a *physical* phenomenon, and physical exercise is one way to "raise" your vibration! Personal trainers would say raise your metabolism, which energetically is the same as raising your vibration.

True magic, the only real form of magic, is *physical* alchemy through the making of decisions and their simultaneous actions. In the case of losing weight, the *only* way to lose weight is to take action, which must include focused exercise. Anything else is just cheating. Anything else is dishonest.

If you learn how to *think* about health and prepare your mind by attaining the right mental state – the right thoughts – health is *very* easy to achieve. In fact, physical health is the *product* of a healthy mental state. When I speak of a healthy mental state, I am not merely talking about the all too familiar cliché, a "positive mental attitude." I am not merely talking about thinking happy thoughts and all will be well. I am saying the true origin of physical health begins at the mental level – in the nonphysical state.

If health were achieved simply by *actions* like eating specific foods, taking certain drugs or supplements, or performing certain exercises, then most of us would be healthy by now. We're not. We are not because we fail to understand that health initiates in the nonphysical mind, the mental state. And *through* physical decisions based on those thoughts, health manifests in the body.

A healthy mental state is a product of having the right thoughts, and the right thoughts are made up of three *acquired* traits: focus, honesty, and awareness, which we will address in the next chapter.

~ 5 ~

FOCUS

Healthy Mental State = FOCUS x Honesty x Awareness

Few of us today really know *how* to focus anymore. We are so easily distracted by technology that it's surprising we can get anything done at all. Creating both the physical environment and the cognitive awareness that facilitate focus can be very challenging. Fortunately, there is an easy way to reacquire this important trait so we can succeed in our own health goals. In some ways, *focus* truly is the easiest of the three acquired traits to develop. But first, let's explore what focus *really* is.

Focus Means Clarity

All of us seem to understand the concept of *focus* as it relates to our ability to see, or when we take a picture. We understand that in order to take a good picture the camera lens must be in focus. Those over 35 years old have all had at one time or another the disappointing experience of getting pictures back from a film developer or digital download only to discover many were not "in focus."

When something isn't in focus, whether it be our vision, a photograph, or even a movie screen, we end up missing out on the full experience. When our vision is out of focus it is difficult to do anything. We can't drive a car, ride a bike, or maybe even walk around our own house! When our vision is out of focus, when the image isn't clear, we often have to slow down. We hesitate. It is because of poor focus that we achieve less than we would if our vision was clear and in focus.

When we use the word *focus* as it relates to the achievement of health goals, the word begins to become a bit more abstract. Why is it some people seem more able than others to achieve their health goals? Why can some people lose weight and get in shape in a month or so and others struggle for years? I contend one of the primary differences between those who achieve easily and those who struggle has to do with this more abstract concept of focus. Focus means having *maximum clarity*. If you want to achieve your health goals you must have maximum clarity of what those goals are.

I often hear people say, "I want to be fit." What does that mean? That's such a generic statement; it's no wonder so few Americans are fit! When someone says to me, "I want to be fit," I ask them to describe for me what they want, *exactly*. Do they have a picture of someone they'd like to look like? Do they have a picture of themselves from an earlier time in their life? Do they know what they would like their measurements to be? Do they want to fit back into a size 32 inch waist pair of jeans? Do they want to fit back into a size 8 dress? What *exactly* do they want to achieve? Focus means a fixed reference point. Do you have an *exact*, fixed reference point for your goals? The following are some examples of focused and unfocused goals.

Focused Goal: "I want to have a 32 inch waist."
Unfocused Goal: "I want to be more fit."

Focused Goal: "I want at least 50% of the food I eat to be organic."
Unfocused Goal: "I want to improve my diet."

Focused Goal: "I want to practice yoga three times a week to relax more."
Unfocused Goal: "I want to have less stress in my life."

Don't Confuse Dreams with Goals

One of the reasons why so many people don't accomplish their goals is because they confuse *dreams* with *goals*. How can you tell the difference between them? Quite simply, *goals* have structure. *Dreams* do not. *Goals* have maximum clarity. *Dreams* are vague. *Goals* can be easily measured in units of some kind and have a timeline. *Dreams* cannot easily be measured. *Goals* are things you are committed to, and you know you are committed to them if you address them *daily*. *Dreams* float in and out of our consciousness haphazardly. I'm not suggesting dreams cannot come true. It's just that a dream can *only* come true if you convert it into a *focused* goal.

Focused goals must be stated in units. What I mean by this is, if you want to lose weight you must measure your weight loss in pounds, clothes sizes or dimensions. If your goal is merely to be "more fit," how are you going to measure progress? If you want to "live a healthier lifestyle," how are you going to measure this? See? You can't measure vague, nonspecific dreams. If you can't *measure* a goal, you can't *achieve* that goal. How would you know if you ever succeeded? Yet most people set unfocused goals that can't be measured. Why is this? Could there be a logical reason for this specificity avoidance? Perhaps there is.

I have often found many people do not really *want* to be any more specific with their goals. This is because being specific can frequently cause pain. Being specific often means a verbal acknowledgment, or even a public acknowledgment, of something currently wrong or unsatisfactory with themselves. Often people do not want to say aloud, "I want to lose my beer gut," or "I want to get rid of all of this cottage cheese on my thighs." They do not want to say these things because saying them simultaneously requires an acknowledgment that the problem exists in the first place! Of course, they already know it's there, but it still hurts to acknowledge it aloud.

You cannot change something like this until you honestly acknowledge its existence. Nothing gets better until you acknowledge aloud and preferably to others that you have a problem, challenge, or goal. I have always

The Honesty Diet

told people: "Health is one of the few things that actually does go away if you ignore it."

Clarity - Knowing Why You Want Something

So many people are obsessed with health goals that do not serve them. For example, I often hear women say they want to lose ten pounds. I then ask them, "Why?"

"Why?" they respond, confused. "Because I want to lose ten pounds, that's why!"

"So," I say, "if you weighed ten pounds less, you'd be happy?"

"That's right."

"OK, let me ask you a question. If I were a genie and I could suddenly grant you your wish of weighing ten pounds less, would you take me up on that?"

"Sure."

"But here's the catch," I say. "Let's say you weigh 150 pounds now, and after I grant you your wish, you'll weigh 140 pounds. However, you won't look any different. All your clothes will fit as they do now. Your face, your hips, legs, rear, and belly will look the same, but you'll have your wish – you will weigh ten pounds less. Would you still be happy?"

"Well... no!"

"Why not?" I ask. "That's what you asked for, isn't it?"

"Why not? Because I won't look any different! Because I won't fit into my clothes properly! Because that isn't at all what I really want!"

Many people strive for goals that are not really what

they want because they haven't ever taken the time to *clarify* exactly what their goals are. You have to really know what your goals are and *why* you want those goals. You also have to recognize what it is you think you'll get from what you say you want.

In the above example, the woman didn't really want to lose ten pounds. What she really wanted was to look better and to fit better into her clothes. Because her thoughts lacked focus, this woman is less likely to achieve what she really wants. By thinking her goal was merely to lose ten pounds, she excluded countless ways of accomplishing her goal. Also, by thinking her goal was merely to lose ten pounds, she may have come up with not-so-healthy ways to accomplish that goal. After all, there are many ways to lose ten pounds. She could choose to become bulimic or anorexic. She could cut off an arm. She could develop cancer. That would certainly help drop the weight. She could dehydrate herself until she weighed ten pounds less.

Without *focus*, without *maximum clarity* of what you want, achieving any health goal can be difficult. It will also frustrate you to expend energy on things you don't really want. To paraphrase something Stephen Covey frequently says in his programs, "It is pretty disappointing to climb all the way to the top of a tall ladder only to discover it is leaning against the wrong wall!"

Frequency – The 2nd Essential Ingredient of Focus

As you can see, clarity is an essential quality of the concept of focus. However, just having maximum clarity of a goal isn't enough. If you set yourself a maximally clarified goal on New Year's Eve, but then stick it in a drawer and never look at it again for the whole year, it is not a focused goal. In the realm of goal achievement, focus is more than just clarity. Focus actually has a second quality… *frequency*.

In order to be focused on a health goal, or any other goal, you must also review and revise that goal on a regular basis. You must review your goal with *maximum frequency*. The more frequently you review your goal, the more committed you will become to that goal. For example, if you review your health goals *daily* (preferably aloud) then you are committed to achieving that goal. If you review your health goals weekly, then you are *kind of* committed to achieving that goal. If you review your health goals *monthly*, then you are *barely* committed to achieving that goal. And, if you review your health goals only *once per year* then you are *not* committed to achieving that goal at all. Therefore, how do you commit to achieving your goals? By increasing the *frequency* with which you review your goals – by reviewing them daily.

*As frequency increases,
commitment increases.*

The Observer Effect

There exists a phenomenon known as the Observer Effect. It is commonly stated like this: The mere *observation* of an event *changes* the event itself. For example, in physics, merely observing an electron with an electron microscope actually changes the trajectory of the electron because the observing light or radiation from the microscope contains enough energy to disturb the location and trajectory of the electron. The same holds true for humans and human behavior because we, of course, are just combinations of trillions of electrons, protons and neutrons.

The Observer Effect can help explain *why when results are measured, results improve*. In general, I believe humans have an innate compulsion to improve their circumstances. It is only when we ignore something that it withers and atrophies. However, when results are measured, one cannot help but to improve those results. For example, when one decides to curtail their spending, often, all that's needed is to become better at *measuring* how much they spend. They may say, "I don't know how to spend less." However, merely measuring their spending, preferably on a daily basis, will often result in their spending less each month. This is because when you do something *daily* it has a tendency to remain in your awareness – in your consciousness. The more frequently you measure, the more likely you are to improve. If you'll just try it, I think you, too, will experience the Observer Effect. You will see how merely measuring an activity subconsciously turns the brain on to improve the outcome.

Like many people, I would set goals around New Year's Eve. Then, at the end of the year I'd review them to see how many I had accomplished. My results weren't that great. Then, a few years ago I simply decided to *measure* my goals more often. At the end of each month, I'd review my progress and set new goals for the following month. Again, I didn't *do* anything differently except I *measured more often*. At the end of the year I was so surprised at how much more I'd accomplished. I almost couldn't believe it! There was no comparison. I had achieved so much more (you might even say 12 times more) than I did by just setting annual goals.

When I decided to measure more often, I didn't necessarily have the foggiest idea *how* I was going to accomplish more at the time, but the process still produced better results. I had tremendous improvement even though reviewing goals merely on a monthly basis certainly isn't being very committed to them.

FOCUS = Clarity x Frequency

Focus is just a product of maximum clarity and frequency. If you don't do these two things, your likelihood for success is minimal.

~ 6 ~

HONESTY

Healthy Mental State = Focus x HONESTY x Awareness

Our trek toward The Honesty Point steepens a bit as we explore the concept of honesty. Don't be frustrated if you notice some more emotional resistance in this chapter.

In addition to *focus*, generating the right thoughts that produce health also requires *honesty*. Honesty is the second acquired trait necessary to possess the healthy mental state. Perhaps, you might not think a health book would include a prominent section on the subject of honesty. Health books tend to focus on subjects such as diet, exercise and stress reduction. In fact, you may not typically think of *honesty* as being a means toward or having anything to do with producing health. But, honesty is, in fact, the very point of this book and is the *key* ingredient to becoming and staying healthy.

When a book discusses *honesty*, you might presume it is a book about relationships and communication, not necessarily health. However, The Honesty Diet *is* about a relationship, and communication within that relationship. It's just the relationship I am referring to is how *honestly* you communicate with yourself. In this chapter, we are going to examine how *honesty* relates to your health and explore what is meant by being *honest* about health. If your doctor said to you, "Be honest with yourself about your health," that wouldn't be a very valuable statement, would it? What does this mean? *How* can we be honest about our health? How do we take a rather abstract and vague concept of *honesty* and relate it in a meaningful way to our health?

Outward Honesty vs. Inward Honesty

When most people think of being honest, they tend to merely think of telling the truth to *others*. This conventional context of honesty is what I call *outward* honesty. Outward honesty is the most basic, most primitive form of honesty. It conveys the notion of telling the truth *to others* like friends, parents, teachers, police officers, judges, employers, etc. Honesty is something we learn at a very young age through classical conditioning – the reward and punishment system. As children, we learn quickly if we say something untrue, we could promptly find ourselves in a heap of trouble, pain, or both.

A second, deeper, and more sophisticated form of honesty exists that isn't commonly taught to us. In fact, it may be something that can't be taught, but something that must be discovered on our own. It is what I call *inward honesty*. Inward honesty is a present and functional awareness of the integrity of one's daily decisions and how congruent they are with one's life values. In the simplest terms, it means being honest with *ourselves*. Inward honesty is a higher, more intelligent form of honesty than outward honesty and is not a trait as easily acquired as outward honesty or focus. Unlike outward honesty, inward honesty requires a preexisting clarity of one's values. We'll learn how to identify our values in a later chapter.

Being inwardly honest requires no formal education, but does require a significant amount of self-reflection. Self-reflection, or self-honesty, is something few of us are good at. We are not very good at it because it isn't something usually taught in school or at home. Sure, we are taught not to lie to others, but rarely are we taught not to lie to *ourselves*.

Outward Dishonesty vs. Inward Dishonesty

Similarly, there are two forms of dishonesty – outward dishonesty and inward dishonesty. Both forms of dishonesty involve pain. However, with outward dishonesty pain is typically inflicted upon us by others, whereas inward dishonesty involves pain inflicted by one's self. And, by pain I don't exclusively mean physical pain. Pain can take many forms, such as embarrassment, the loss of opportunity, or the loss of self-respect.

With outward dishonesty, we are usually able to associate and determine a cause-and-effect relationship.

We are consciously aware of dishonesty at the time of its telling. For example, a young girl eats some cookies from the kitchen pantry after being told not to by a parent. When caught, the little girl professes to the parent that she did not eat any cookies. The child is well aware she is lying. There is a deliberate attempt to deceive and a conscious effort to avoid the taking of responsibility and incurring the associated consequence.

With inward dishonesty, we may or may not be aware of being dishonest at the time of its telling depending on what level of awareness we possess at that time. The effects or pain of a lie we tell ourselves, especially as it pertains to our health, may not necessarily be evident for years or even decades. For example, we may drink alcohol daily believing it is good for our cardiovascular health only to discover it later contributed to adult onset diabetes, high blood pressure, and liver cirrhosis. However, if we were really being honest and paying attention to our health, we easily could have recognized that drinking alcohol daily wasn't good for us.

Through this book, we are going to learn to boldly acknowledge dishonesty – that is, address when we are lying to and cheating ourselves. We will learn to recognize self-honesty as a source of freedom and choice, and dishonesty as a source of pain and imprisonment. "But I am honest," you say. "I don't lie to myself." Actually, I contend all of us at times lie to ourselves. I do not exclude myself from this affliction.

Layers of Honesty

There are many layers and levels of honesty that we have the opportunity to transcend – to move beyond – every day of our lives. What may be honest on one level of awareness isn't necessarily honest on a higher level of awareness, or vice versa. Through a genuine use of inward honesty, we have the opportunity to recognize over time something we once thought was honest, no longer is.

The opposite may also be true. For example, eating energy bars may seem healthy to a person at one level of awareness, but may later be recognized as unhealthy when that persons shifts to a higher level of awareness. What determines whether or not something is honest or dishonest is how that something relates to our values and our acknowledgment (or lack of acknowledgment) of those values. The evolution of inward honesty is similar to the peeling of an onion. There's always another layer.

There is nothing wrong with discovering we are being dishonest with ourselves. Quite the contrary, every time we discover, acknowledge, and embrace the fact that we have been dishonest with ourselves on some level, it creates an opportunity. We create an opportunity to grow, to become more healthy, to become happier and more fulfilled, and to become more successful. *Our ability to be honest with ourselves yields the power to control and direct our lives consciously.* Our ability to be honest with ourselves is limited only by our level of consciousness or awareness.

Don't Spend Your Health Earning Wealth

I am always amazed at how many people spend their *health* early in life trying to earn *wealth*, only to discover later they must spend all of their hard-earned *wealth* trying to regain their *health*. What's more, they fail to make the connection between the two. After all, what good is being wealthy and dead? Many people think this life path is normal – that it is normal to earn and save money their whole working life so they can spend it treating their cancer or heart disease in retirement.

In the United States things have gotten so bad it's almost as though "retirement" is a synonym for "disease treatment" – the treatment of diseases they developed while working. Americans think it's normal to grow old in their 50s, to become sick in their 60s and die in their 70s! While this may be very common in the United States, it certainly isn't normal!

People who fit this profile were not being honest with themselves. In fact, they were being quite inwardly dishonest. Their priorities simply weren't in order because they failed to have an inwardly honest dialogue with themselves. They thought they could cheat and get away with it. As they pursued their careers and as they raised their families, they thought their bodies didn't need adequate sleep, nutritious foods, and regular exercise to mitigate stress. They felt they "didn't have time" for these things. Their bodies compensated as best they could for a while. But eventually their decisions caught up to them, in the form of a life-threatening disease, such as cancer, heart disease, obesity or diabetes.

Learning to Recognize Truth

Inward honesty can be better understood when discussed in a context of relationships. For example, let's say a bride suddenly leaves a groom at the altar or breaks off an engagement. A perception may exist among others that she was afraid of commitment and got cold feet. Rarely is such an action thought to be an action of inward honesty. But, isn't it possible her sudden and seemingly erratic decision was really a manifestation of honesty toward her internal feelings – an internal truth coming to the surface? Could this not be a completely rational and reasonable attempt to avoid making a costly mistake? Could this not be an expression of inward honesty?

When you learn to be honest with yourself, everything else in life begins to become much easier. Unfortunately, learning to be more honest is not a singular event. Honesty, and the awareness that follows, presents itself not all at once, but over time and experience. It is a process that must be practiced daily.

Do We Really Want the Truth?

Truth is an interesting notion given much attention throughout human history. Truth was an especially popular idea of exploration by philosophers, such as Socrates, Aristotle, and Immanuel Kant. Indeed, the acknowledgment of truth may be the entire aim of the human condition.

> *"Men occasionally stumble over the truth, but most of them pick themselves up and hurry off as if nothing ever happened."*
> – Sir Winston Churchill

I suggest the reason we "hurry off" from truth as in the Churchill quote above, is because we don't like the honest truth, and because we don't, we just ignore it. In my opinion, we already know nearly *all* the answers to obtaining and maintaining good health – we just don't *like* those answers. So we ignore the truth and keep on looking for answers that please us and make us feel comfortable or not responsible for the negative things we experience. For example, you may elect to begin a fad diet, one that recommends eliminating virtually all carbohydrates and replacing them with greasy, fat-laden meats. You know in your gut this doesn't make sense, but you choose to go on the diet anyway because deep down you love the magical notion that eating greasy, fast-food burgers can help you to lose weight.

Don't Take Advice From Fat Doctors!

Every few months we hear on the news about a new study which has discovered some vice of ours actually has an alleged "health" benefit. For example, eating chocolate is good for you because it contains antioxidants, important nutrients for anti-aging. Drinking coffee decreases the risk of colon cancer. Or, drinking beer decreases the development of cataracts. What these news stories fail to tell you is that fruits and vegetables contain antioxidants, but don't make you fat, don't contribute to diabetes, and don't ruin your complexion, which makes them a far healthier choice. Drinking water also decreases your risk of colon cancer without affecting your sleep function and hormone levels the way coffee does. And, fruits and vegetables will also decrease your risk of developing cataracts without causing you to crash your car or develop a beer belly. Whenever these "pop-culture" studies emerge, they only encourage us to continue to be dishonest with ourselves about our health.

The Churchill quote reminds me of another funny story illustrating how we often ignore truth and pretend to continue to search for more pleasant, comforting answers.

> An old man is in a parking lot one night looking for his dropped car keys beneath a street light. A young lady walks up and says, "Can I help you with something?"
> "I dropped my car keys," he responds.
> "Oh, my. May I help you look for them?"
> "Thanks. That would be wonderful." After a few minutes of searching the young lady says,

"I don't see them anywhere! Where do you think you dropped them?"

"Way over there," the old man says, pointing to the far, dark end of the parking lot.

"Well, if you dropped them over there, why are you looking for them over here?"

"Because over here is where the light is!"

How Do We Learn to Think Honestly?

Psychologists have proposed that *thinking* is simply the process of asking and answering questions to oneself. If this is the case, then perhaps the reason we as a society have lost our ability to *think* about health is because we have lost the habit of asking ourselves questions about health.

Today we rarely try to solve a health issue by ourselves because that would require too much work – and, of course, we are *far* too busy with more important things, like our children's sports activities, television, and shopping. We would rather pay a doctor to give us an answer, even though she may not necessarily give us the right answer. Indeed then, it is our *laziness* as a society – our unwillingness to think – that makes us so unhealthy.

To regain your ability to *think* about health, you have to begin the process of *honestly* asking and answering questions to yourself about health. The following is an exercise meant to catalyze the process of reacquiring this suppressed innate ability to *think*. I recommend asking what I call "context-negative" questions because I believe they help stimulate thinking by pointing out the absurdity of one's current actions or thinking patterns. Take a good look at all the things you do on a daily basis, and based on your daily choices and actions, begin to ask yourself *honest* questions like these:

- Do you *honestly* think the reason you're so tired in the morning is because you *don't* have enough caffeine in your bloodstream?
- Do you *honestly* think the reason you have so many cavities in your mouth is because there *isn't* enough fluoride on your teeth?
- Do you *honestly* think the reason your energy levels spike and crash throughout the day is because you're not eating enough "energy" bars?
- Do you *honestly* think the reason you have so many aches and pains is because there *isn't* enough pain killer medication in your bloodstream?
- Do you *honestly* think the reason you might struggle with depression is because there isn't enough antidepressant drug in your body?
- Do you *honestly* think the reason your child can't concentrate in class is because he doesn't have enough narcotic-like drugs (ADD/ADHD medication) in his bloodstream?
- Do you *honestly* think the reason you are so overweight is because you aren't eating enough diet foods or drinking enough diet sodas? Or because your stomach isn't properly stapled shut (gastric bypass surgery)?

The Honesty Diet

- Do you *honestly* think the reason you are so overweight is because you eat *too many* fresh fruits and vegetables?
- Do you *honestly* think the reason why your clothes don't fit like they used to is because the dry cleaner shrunk them?
- Do you *honestly* think the reason you have trouble going to the bathroom with any regularity is because you consume *too much* fiber?
- Do you *honestly* think the best way to avoid breast cancer is to surgically cut off your breasts? Along that same logic, do you think, then, the best way to avoid *brain* cancer is to cut out your *brain*?

Facetiousness Elucidates Honesty

I know some of these context-negative questions may sound facetious, but they really do illustrate the limited extent to which many people *think* about their health. One person who read these questions thought I was trying to be funny. But the truth is, I wasn't. How many times have you heard someone say, "Sorry, I'm a bit out of it today. I haven't had my coffee, yet." As if the real reason they're tired is because they don't have enough caffeine in their system!

Use your brain. *Think*. Ask and answer questions *honestly*. Do these kinds of questions make sense? Of course, they don't. Yet these are precisely some of the ways in which many people try to address their health. Be *honest*. The fact of the matter is we all already know the answers to most of our health problems. We simply don't like the honest answers – we don't like the truth. So we seek out dishonest answers that keep us from having to change.

Let's explore some of these questions one at a time.

Do you honestly think the reason you're so tired in the morning is because you don't have enough caffeine in your bloodstream?

Honestly, why do you think you're tired in the morning? Is it because you've convinced yourself you are just not a morning person? No, not if you're being honest. Are you the kind of person who says, "I only need five to six hours of sleep per night," but then you consume ten to twenty cups of coffee each day? Why do you *think* you're so tired in the morning? Might it be because you don't *value* sleep? Do you lie in bed watching television for hours before going to sleep? Do you fall asleep with the TV on? Are you on your bright screen computer until late at night? Do you go to bed close to midnight and get up for work at 5 a.m.? Do you watch the violent news an hour before bed? Do you have to drink alcoholic beverages in the evening to relax and calm yourself down so you can fall asleep?

Furthermore, do you think caffeine is naturally found in the body? No, of course, not. Then why do you *behave* as if the reason you're so tired in the morning is because you don't have enough of a chemical in your body you know shouldn't be there in the first place? What is the first thing you do in the morning? Do you stumble into the kitchen and guzzle your morning jug of coffee? Is it possible you could wake up your body gradually by, oh, I don't know, maybe *moving* it! You know, like by doing some modest exercise. Honestly, the only reason why you are tired in the morning is because you don't *choose* to get a good night's sleep. You lie to yourself and say you only need a few hours, but that isn't true. If it were true, you wouldn't drink coffee.

Do you honestly think the reason you have so many cavities is because there isn't enough fluoride on your teeth?

The issue of fluoride is a controversial one. Many credible groups and individuals claim fluoride is safe and helps prevent tooth decay. Many equally credible groups and individuals claim fluoride cannot be said to be safe, and they can point to research suggesting it may be linked to a number of diseases including cancer, hypothyroidism, and Down's syndrome. This book will not explore this highly controversial issue. However, one should ask, *honestly*, is it natural to spike water sources with a highly reactive chemical substance that doesn't naturally exist in the body in the first place?

Do you honestly think the reason you have so many aches and pains is because there isn't enough pain killer medication in your bloodstream?

People tend to ignore things like joint pain and its valuable message by covering the pain up with drugs. In fact, our society conditions us to *ignore* pain. Men are taught to ignore pain because men should "tough it out." Women learn that pain is *normal* because they suffer monthly with their menstrual periods. Neither belief is true or healthy, but each gender learns that life is pain. The result is we ignore the culprits that cause us pain. We eat junk food, which erodes our joints and joint tissues. We choose not to sleep well, which prevents our joints from healing. We tend to be sedentary, which atrophies our joints and muscles. Then, instead of fixing the problems we know are actually *causing* our pain, we *choose* to take drugs that don't heal us but merely chemically prevent our brain from feeling the pain. We then go about our business as if the problem's solved.

I saw a television commercial for a pain-relieving drug reinforcing this damaging thought process. The commercial portrayed a baby-boomer-age woman who wanted to dance, but couldn't because her knees hurt too much from chronic arthritis. However, after she took some magical over-the-counter pain-reliever she could dance all night long. The commercial ends with her spinning across the dance floor smiling.

What is really happening here? Are her knees suddenly "better" after taking the medication? Did they miraculously heal? No. In fact, the drug didn't affect her knees at all. It only convinced her brain there was no pain. No pain meant she could dance, right? Well, what happens when the drug wears off? Are her knees *healthier* now than they were before she took the pain reliever? Not if we're being honest, they're not. In fact, her knees are probably worse now than they were before taking the drug. There is most likely *more* damage now, after dancing the night away, than there was before.

She didn't listen to the message her knees were sending her. The pain in her knees was sending her a message that she shouldn't dance *right now*. The pain was meant to limit her mobility while her knees tried to heal. She didn't care, though. She thought she could tell her knees what to do and how to feel. By taking drugs, she may be temporarily pain-free, but the relief won't last. If she had just taken the time to let her knees heal, she may have had decades more of dancing. But if she continues to ignore her body's messages, covering them up with drugs, she isn't likely to be dancing at all much longer.

We all know how dangerous it can be to combine alcohol with prescription drugs. Well, combining dishonesty with pharmaceutical drugs can also be extremely dangerous. I knew someone who had headaches every single day for over a year. Instead of looking into the *cause* of the headache, he took a common over-the-counter pain reliever daily instead. One day, he noticed some purple splotching on his feet. He didn't think much of it. A few days later the blotches had spread over his entire body. He went to the hospital where it was determined he was bleeding internally throughout his entire body.

Why? Because this "safe" over-the-counter medication so many people take regularly had virtually shut down his spleen. The medication "works" by reducing the clotting mechanism involved in the production of pain and inflammation. By masking his pain with this so-called safe medication, he almost internally bled to death.

This is just one example of what can happen when you're not being honest with yourself and just try to cover up your problems with drugs.

~ 7 ~

AWARENESS

Healthy Mental State = Focus x Honesty x AWARENESS

Awareness is the third component of cultivating the good thoughts that produce good health. Good thoughts *originate* from a specific level of awareness. And, this specific level of awareness cannot be achieved without engaging in a *focused* self-dialogue of deep, straightforward *honesty*.

Awareness can be an ambiguous term. For some people, awareness means increasing public awareness for a societal message – such as an environmental cause like a "Save the Whales" campaign. For others, *raising awareness* conjures up metaphysical imagery complete with "airy-fairy" spiritual connotations. By itself, the word *aware* simply means "paying attention." But, when the word *awareness* is used, its meaning becomes less clear.

In recent years the words *awareness* and *consciousness* have taken on a meta-physical context. Entire sections of bookstores have even been dedicated to the exploration of the relationship of awareness and consciousness to spiritual evolution. This, I think, has soured many to the concept of awareness. While I do not necessarily challenge this relationship, from a daily, practical use standpoint, it isn't required to learn how to raise your level of awareness. You simply don't need to become a guru, yogi master, samurai, Jedi knight or practice any kind of meditation to live life at a higher level of awareness.

Let's attempt to simplify *awareness* into a more useful, workable concept, particularly as it relates to health.

The term *awareness* has been defined as "knowledge gained through one's perception." Awareness suggests a higher than average acuity – a mental acuity. It means a better way of thinking or a better way of *mentally perceiving* any given situation. That's quite different from the basic meaning of the word aware – "paying attention." Sometimes raising awareness is also referred to as raising one's *consciousness*. For the intents and purposes of this book, the terms raising one's *awareness* and raising one's *consciousness* are interchangeable. However, for simplicity, we will refer to this concept as raising *awareness*. The following examples may help illustrate the term awareness in this book.

The Honesty Diet

Hidden in Plain Sight

Have you ever seen those 3-D images, called autostereograms? Upon first glance it appears to look like a random pattern of lines and colors, but as you look at it more closely, relax your gaze and allow your eyes to adjust, a floating three-dimensional object gradually becomes visible *within* the art?

Some say the image is "hidden" in the art, but in fact, the image isn't hidden at all. Rather, it's quite large and positioned right smack in the middle of the artwork. It's just most people will not *perceive* the image as being there unless they have been made *aware* of its existence beforehand. A person may, in fact, be "aware" in the simplest sense that they are paying attention to the art, but only if they actually *raise* their awareness of what is *within* the art will they eventually "see" the image right in front of them.

Another example of awareness could be illustrated this way: Take a publicly-traded company's stock chart. To many people, looking at a stock chart is very much like looking at ancient Greek. Even though they may be *aware* of the stock chart (they are looking *at* it), and although they may be paying attention to it, the chart may not make much sense. Therefore, that person is said to have a low level of *awareness* about that chart. But with a little *education* and an *honest* willingness to learn, they can dramatically raise their level of awareness. They'll not just learn how to read a stock chart, but will come to understand how a stock chart can benefit them – by making them a lot of money, perhaps. So, awareness is raised when a thing is given *more meaning*.

Awareness is giving more meaning to something.

"The problems of today cannot be solved at the same *level of thinking* that existed when the problem was created." In Einstein's famous quote, the same *level of thinking* is another way of saying *awareness*. "The problems of today cannot be solved at the same *awareness* that existed when the problem was created." Awareness is a level of thinking. Higher levels of thinking mean higher levels of awareness. The question then is *how* does one raise their awareness?

Raising One's Health Awareness

Let's apply this simplified understanding of awareness to a health example. Most people know they *should* get a good night's sleep, but statistics show about two-thirds of Americans *choose* not to. However, when you educate them that a good night's sleep isn't just a good idea so they'll have enough energy for the next day. It also rejuvenates the immune system, balances emotional health, and helps to lose body fat. Sleep now undertakes *more meaning* for that person. Sleep now has more *significance* and *value*, and immediate benefits which can be gained from this knowledge. If they had then taken action on such information, they would have *raised awareness* about the value of getting a good night's sleep.

Previously, they knew they *should* get a good night's sleep, but they didn't necessarily know *why* they should. They did not know because they had a lower *awareness* of the value of sleep. But now they have a higher awareness than they did before. Perhaps you do, too. Perhaps you did not know, until just now, that quality sleep helps you lose body fat, balance emotions, and rejuvenate your immune system. If you now *act* upon this education, you will have raised your awareness.

Acknowledging Ignorance

Raising one's awareness is not always easy. In order to learn something new, we must first acknowledge to ourselves, and often to others, that we don't understand something. Admitting, "I don't know" can be rather difficult – for some it can even be embarrassing. Why? Because from kindergarten through high school and college we were rewarded for answering questions correctly and penalized for answering questions incorrectly. We were conditioned to try to get the answers right even if we had to guess. Surely, we've all been snickered at by classmates because we didn't know the right answer to an easy question, or because we just got the answer wrong. Inside, we are still that same kid, with the same fear of being laughed at. We're just bigger now.

Increasing Awareness Can Cause Pain

At least in the short run, raising awareness can be an unattractive and sometimes painful process for some. Raising awareness requires being *honest* with yourself, which is often extremely difficult to do. For example, many people live month-to-month financially. This is often because they have a low level of *financial awareness*. Financial awareness isn't the same thing as financial education. Financial awareness means you are educated *and honest* about your financial circumstances.

For those who live month-to-month, consciously recognizing they are living beyond their means can be the most painful thing they've ever done. Often, people discover they could not even survive the slightest financial hiccup. Acknowledging this can be even more painful than simply ignoring the situation and continuing to live month to month. But, when that financial hiccup or worse comes along, they then wish they hadn't ignored their circumstances for so long. For these people, financial *education*, by itself without inward honesty, isn't likely to help.

The same thing holds true for one's health. If you live your life at a very low level of *health awareness*, you, too, will likely find yourself in a lot of trouble sooner or later. And, just as with financial awareness, merely increasing health education usually will not help. You must first raise your awareness by practicing self-honesty about your health. Following a diet that contends it is healthy to eliminate an entire source of food like carbohydrates, fats or protein would be one example of living life at a low level of health awareness. Anyone practicing honesty should plainly see this simply isn't a healthy practice. There is an innate awareness within each of us that inherently knows a diet model like this simply doesn't make sense. Ultimately, such a belief, such a low level of awareness, will harm you.

What's the Payoff?

So, why would you want to raise your awareness, especially if becoming aware can be painful? What does raising your awareness do for you? Why should you strive for it? The benefit of raising your awareness, of perceiving things with more acuity, *with more meaning,* than you have in the past, is this: A higher awareness provides greater and better options in life and health. More options mean more freedom. And, generally speaking, the more freedom you have, be it physical freedom, financial freedom, or emotional freedom, the healthier and higher quality of life you can have.

The higher your awareness climbs, the higher the quality of your thoughts. The higher quality thoughts you have, the better decisions you will make to produce and maintain health. These better decisions, once again, raise your awareness. Indeed, it is a self-perpetuating health cycle.

Five Powerful Words

Years ago, I learned what I think are the five most powerful words in the world. Those words are: "*What makes you say that?*" It is through these words that I came to realize how often we believe things, think things, or assume things to be true that aren't necessarily so. These five simple words are a great tool for raising awareness.

For example, years before I became a doctor, I went to a physician's office for a visit. In the waiting room on the table were several health magazines. While browsing through one of them, I came across an article about a parent who chose not to vaccinate her children. A parent who *didn't* vaccinate her children, I thought? It must be some mistake. Why would a parent not vaccinate her children? While visiting with the doctor, I brought up the subject. I foolishly proclaimed, "I think it is irresponsible to not vaccinate your child."

"*What makes you say that?*" she said.

"Well... because! Vaccines prevent children from getting various diseases!"

"*What makes you say that?*" she said again.

"What makes me say that? Everybody knows that! Your children would get sick and die without them."

"*What makes you say that?*" she repeated for a third time.

"Well, ummm... because, they would, that's why! You know, herd-immunity, that sort of thing."

She paused and said, "I chose not to vaccinate my daughter, and I know she is healthier for it."

Oh, crap. I thought to myself.

"May I ask you a few questions?" she continued.

The Honesty Diet

"Sure," I said, while trying to take the foot out of my mouth.

"Do you know what chemical ingredients are in vaccines?"

"No."

"Do you know who makes vaccines?"

"I'm not sure."

"Can you tell me how many children have been permanently injured or killed by vaccines?"

"No, I can't."

"I just asked you three simple questions about vaccines you couldn't answer, yet you seem to be adamantly defending your *belief* that it is irresponsible to not vaccinate your children. Tell me, do think it is *intelligent* – do you think it is responsible – to adamantly defend things you, by your own admission, clearly know absolutely nothing about? Does that make sense to you?"

"No," I said, defeated. "I guess, not."

The point of this story is not to tell you whether or not you should vaccinate your children. That is up to you. The point is to beware of an unquestioned conviction. So many of us have strong health beliefs, religious beliefs, political beliefs, and social beliefs, but we have no idea why we believe them. We've never explored them with any level of *honesty* or *thinking*. Many of these beliefs and opinions were programmed into us by parents, teachers, doctors, religions, friends and employers, even though they may bear no relation to reality whatsoever.

Learning to say either to ourselves or to others, "What makes you say that?" is a tool which can help raise awareness and teach us to think again. By once again learning how to think for ourselves, we can make conscious choices about our health – to not just be programmed robots living our lives by society's social norms and expectations.

Here's another set of powerful, magical words: *"How's that working for you?"* If the answer is "It isn't," then perhaps you need to reexamine that belief, that approach, or that method. For example, a grad school classmate of mine wanted to lose some weight. He decided to try a popular diet which advocated eating tons of meat and doesn't emphasize fruits and vegetables. After a couple of months, I asked him, "How's that working for you?"

"Not so good," he said. "I've actually gained about ten pounds."

"Maybe that fad diet isn't the right approach for you," I offered.

"No. I really like it. I'm going to stick with it."

He never lost the weight. He just became fatter because he wasn't being honest with himself. The popular diet was attractive to him, because he felt it allowed him to eat lots of fat, greasy foods he enjoyed. However, he gained weight. It simply wasn't a very honest way of approaching weight loss. He was approaching his weight problem from a highly dishonest perspective.

Learning to ask yourself, *"How's that working for you?"* can be another effective tool for evaluating whether or not something you are doing is honestly serving you or not.

How Education and Honesty Relate

We in the United States are familiar with trying to raise awareness through *education*. In fact, you could say our whole society is obsessed with education. We seem to think almost every problem – environmental problems, social problems, you name it – can be solved through more education. I don't necessarily disagree with this. Education is important. But, education without honesty is futile.

How valuable education is depends upon whether or not you are being honest. I propose what we really lack isn't enough education, but enough honesty. Indeed, people are often over-educated, but under-honest with themselves, in that getting *more* education doesn't necessarily mean improving their circumstances without their first being more honest with themselves.

For example, two of the biggest and most common problems Americans face are 1) health problems, and 2) financial problems. It is common that health problems often *cause* financial problems. It is equally common that financial problems often cause health problems. The two bear an intimate relationship to one another. On the other hand, people rarely have political science problems, art history problems, or English literature problems. Yet, it is often subjects like these people *focus* on in high school and college. It seems to me if health problems and financial problems are the two biggest areas of concern for adults, perhaps it is *these* subjects we should be focusing our education on, not English literature, art history, or political science. Yet, primary education doesn't thoroughly teach subjects like health and personal finance.

I'm not dismissing the value of a rounded education. But I do believe we have our priorities mixed up. *Honestly, do you think the reason why you have health problems today is because you didn't study enough political science in school?* Certainly, not. However, do you think it is possible you have health problems today because you didn't learn *how* to be healthy earlier in life? Probably, so. It is well recognized that most cases of heart disease, cancer, and obesity can be avoided if we simply *choose* to live properly.

Why didn't most people learn to be healthy in elementary school, high school or college? It is because, overwhelmingly, Americans have traditionally outsourced the maintenance of their health to doctors. We've been brainwashed since childhood to believe we can do whatever we want to our bodies, and it is the doctor's job to "fix" whatever ails us with drugs, surgery, or supplements when the body breaks down. I find it ironic that so many Americans today are upset over American companies outsourcing labor to cheaper foreign countries, but seem to have no problem with outsourcing for over 100 years the maintenance of our health to doctors.

Am I suggesting we all should study medicine? No, I'm not. *Medicine* does not make us healthy. Medicine only keeps us alive in emergency situations. If medicine made us healthy, then it would stand to reason that medical physicians would be one of the healthiest groups of people in the country. To the best of my knowledge, there is no indication this is the case. The truth is doctors often have just as many health problems as non-doctors and use just as many drugs (in some cases more) as non-doctors. I contend this is because many doctors do not understand health at its root. Overwhelmingly, most doctors are still being trained to study *disease*, not *health*. Subsequently, they practice what they were taught – disease treatment instead of health promotion. These, of course, are not the same things.

The Limits of Education

We must recognize that without *honesty*, education has limited value. For example, let's say you are a smoker and you really would like to avoid developing lung cancer, but you're not willing to give up smoking. So you go get *educated* on lung cancer. You read and learn everything you can about lung cancer. You even learn more than most doctors know about lung cancer. Without a doubt, through education, you have raised your awareness to some extent about lung cancer and the adverse effects of smoking. The only problem is… you still smoke!

Despite everything you have learned about lung cancer, you still haven't quit the behavior causing lung cancer. Why? You weren't being *honest* with yourself. The only reason you studied lung cancer was to try to find a way to avoid developing it *without having to quit smoking*. Sounds ridiculous, right? Of course, it does. That is because your approach was dishonest. Trying to avoid lung cancer without quitting smoking seems pretty stupid. Obviously, the best thing to do to avoid developing lung cancer is to not smoke. Your intent of raising your awareness through education wasn't motivated by an *honest* effort to be healthy. Instead, you became educated on lung cancer in an effort to cheat, or to get around having to quit smoking.

I know this example may seem a bit silly. Perhaps you think this is a rather unrealistic scenario – that most people would know they have to stop smoking to prevent lung cancer and heart disease. Still, I would contend this scenario isn't all that silly. In fact, people do exactly this every day in other areas of life and health. Let's go through this example again. But this time we are going to change the scenario, just a bit, to see whether or not it is really that unrealistic.

Let's say, instead, you eat like a pig, are overweight, and you would really like to be thin and fit. So you go get *educated* on several different diet programs. You read and learn everything there is to know about dieting. You are so thorough, you even end up learning more than most health professionals know about the subject. Without a doubt, through education, you have raised your awareness to some extent about dieting and weight loss. The only problem is... you still eat like a pig! Despite everything you have learned about diets and weight loss, you still haven't changed the behavior making you overweight. Why? Again, I propose it's because you weren't being honest with yourself. I suggest the only reason you studied diet and weight loss was to try to find a way to not be overweight without having to stop eating like a pig and eating things that make you fat.

Does this *still* sound ridiculous? Isn't this exactly what most people do? You see, without *honesty*, education can only take us so far. We must, therefore, learn to be honest with ourselves *before* making any efforts to increase our education.

The reason the smoking scenario seems so ridiculous is because in the United States there already exists a *cultural awareness*, or a *societal truth*, that smoking causes lung cancer and heart disease. It is well known and well accepted by the overwhelming majority of the population that the best way to prevent lung cancer and other related adverse conditions is to not smoke. However, the cultural awareness that the best way to lose weight and be fit is to *not eat like a pig* doesn't exist yet, even though it is just as true as the smoking awareness. Sure, some people understand this, but the overwhelming majority of Americans still deny it.

In this country eating like a pig is perceived as something to be proud of. Have you seen fast-food television ads for things like giant cheeseburgers? A few friends go out for a burger, fries, and a soda. We then see them sweating, beading at the forehead, wiping their brow, almost passing out as they painstakingly try to consume this massive amount of fast-food. The ad creates the perception of an achievement worthy of praise and respect to eat this quantity of food. It's almost daring you to try. It is no wonder we are so fat! The image of the "American Pig" is idolized by our society.

Most Americans still believe they can healthfully lose weight and be fit by eating "energy" bars, drinking meal replacement shakes and diet colas, and by eliminating entire food sources like carbohydrates from the diet. Americans are overweight because they simply eat too much bad stuff and not enough good stuff. It's just that simple. That is the *honest* answer. I contend that the weight loss example above is just as true and realistic as the smoking example, but it may not seem that way to many because the country's *societal awareness* simply hasn't yet evolved to a level of acknowledgment that eating like a pig *causes* obesity. If it had, then no one would be purchasing all of those fad diet books, diet products, fat-burning supplements, and fat-burning gizmos we all see advertised on television.

The Primary Cause of Obesity, Poor Health and Most Disease

All this talk about focus, honesty, and awareness has been leading to my main assertion. I firmly contend the *fundamental* cause of obesity, poor health, and most disease in the United States is *dishonesty*. This is a belief, not necessarily a provable assertion. However, by the time you are finished reading this book, I trust you will understand what I mean by dishonesty and how by applying this insight will significantly improve your health and quality of life.

When people are not honest with themselves about their health, their careers, and their relationships, they set the stage for actions – the conscious and unconscious choices – ultimately manifesting as poor health and disease. A person suffering from a chronic disease may never identify dishonesty as the cause of their physical

The Honesty Diet

problems, problems that could eventually take their life without the person ever recognizing dishonesty as its cause.

*Chronic dishonesty causes chronic disease.
Chronic honesty causes chronic health.*

Answer this question: Which organ of the body is most closely associated with the experience of *honesty*? I bet most of you would say the heart. Some will say the gut. But either way, we associate honesty with these organs. The heart and/or the gut are the *organs of honesty*. In language we say, "I know *in my heart*" that something is true. Or, we say, "I know I'm right about this. I feel it *in my gut.*" When someone says something is coming *from the heart*, they mean they're being brutally honest, straightforward, and down to earth. If I am correct that the fundamental cause of obesity, poor health, and most disease is dishonesty, isn't it interesting that heart disease and colon (gut) cancer are two of the biggest killers in the United States? Is it possible our long-lived, chronic dishonesty with ourselves manifests – through our daily choices – as diseases like heart disease or colon cancer? To understand *how* this occurs, refer back to the formula we started with at the beginning of this book.

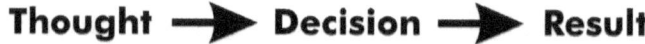

Thought ➔ Decision ➔ Result

Dishonest *thoughts* produce dishonest decisions. Over time, dishonest decisions manifest in our bodies. The *result* is obesity, pain, poor health and/or physical disease. Consider the following story:

> During her primary education, a young woman never learns about the true origins of health. She does not learn to create good health. She does not learn to maintain it. She does not learn to be honest about health, which means she has low health awareness. In adulthood, she *chooses* to focus her full attention on her fast-growing career, at the expense of her health. She chooses to forego adequate sleep, proper nutrition, exercise, and stress reduction for a period of 20+ years so she can "get ahead" in life.
>
> During these 20 years she *chooses* to marry and have children. Now, because she's even busier, she *chooses* to use her marriage and children as another excuse not to focus on her health. When she begins to have digestive problems like gastric reflux, instead of being *honest* and *choosing* to make healthful lifestyle changes, she ignores her body's messages and, instead, *chooses* to cover them up with a prescription drug. That drug causes other problems in her body, so she *chooses* to take a second drug to address the side effects of the first drug. Because she *chooses* not to focus on her health, her children are also deprived of proper nutrition, restful sleep, and regular exercise.
>
> Within a few years, both of her boys are "suddenly" diagnosed with Attention Deficit

The Honesty Diet

Hyperactivity Disorder and Mom *chooses* to start giving them prescription narcotic-like drugs to cover up their alleged illness. Over time, when the prescription drugs and medical insurance premiums progressively increase, they begin to take a toll on the family's finances. Medical expenses impact the family's budget so much so that she *chooses* to put in an additional 15 hours per week at work, just to make ends meet.

The added stress from the additional hours at work puts even more stress than there already was on her marriage. After six more months of this, her husband files for divorce. After the divorce, the woman's expenses increase again, because not only is she awarded primary custody of the kids, but she is now, for the most part, surviving only on one income. She handles the additional stress by choosing to eat more, and rapidly gains weight. Now her clothes don't fit. There's another expense.

A few years later, she is tired, achy and ill all the time, and can't understand why and in spite of the drugs, the children's ADHD still hasn't "gone away." She also doesn't understand why one of her sons – who has now been taking prescription drugs for years – has started experimenting with recreational drugs. She becomes depressed, and instead of addressing her body's needs she again covers up the problem by taking antidepressant medication. She decides she needs a vacation to "recharge." She goes to a Mexico resort for a week and drinks herself into a stupor to forget all her problems back home. When

Don't Take Advice From Fat Doctors!

she returns home, the drinking continues. Within a few months she loses her job, because she is no longer a productive employee. With her job also goes the medical insurance benefits. A year later, she starts having heart and circulation difficulties. She goes to her doctor who informs her that she has heart disease and he's found a cancerous lump in one of her breasts. Stunned, she asks her doctor, *"Why did this happen to me?"*

The doctor shrugs his shoulders and says, "I'm sorry. It's genetic. There's nothing you could have done to prevent it. I strongly recommend we perform a radical mastectomy and begin radiation and/or chemotherapy right away. It's your best chance for survival."

Even more depressed now, the woman goes home drops to her knees and asks God, "I have so many problems already, why did *you* do this to me?" As a result of the costs of her medical treatment, she *chooses* to prematurely redeem her 401K nest egg to pay for the ongoing medical expenses and support herself during her "sudden" illness. After a year of treatment, she is bald, but in remission for now, and *chooses* to work at a supercenter retail store making minimum wage as a cashier.

Although this fictitious story is a bit extreme, it is an attempt to illustrate the cascade of events – of *choices* we make or choices we *don't* make – ultimately determining our health. This is an example of a woman who spent her health trying to accumulate wealth, to get ahead,

The Honesty Diet

who in the end had to spend her wealth trying to regain her health (and not very successfully). Can you see how this woman's experiences and predicament was not a function of things that happened to her, but a product of her dishonesty and the dishonest choices she made *every step along the way to disaster*? She took her health for granted. She failed to put her priorities in order. And, when she was diagnosed with cancer she still denied it had something to do with her *choices*, and instead blamed God for her troubles. I'll bet you know someone with something close to this experience. Perhaps, it is even your experience.

~ 8 ~

LANGUAGE LIES

Political Correctness and Language Lies

The next leg of our journey increases in difficulty once again as we explore the concept of language lies.

> *"Is a man's man now called a person's person?"*
>
> – Comedian, George Carlin

Political correctness is a societal effort to eliminate social bias within language. For example, at the time of this writing, in the United States the most common example of political correctness may be the use of the term "African American" instead of "black." In recent decades, this linguistic phenomenon has taken our country by storm. Overall, I think political correctness has benefited society, particularly in the way people often refer to others of different cultures, persuasions and ethnicity. Generally, being politically correct does not hurt anyone and is considered to be polite and appropriate behavior. Political correctness comes in very handy when dealing with others under difficult circumstances, when we can replace painful words with softer ones. For example, when someone dies, we often choose to soften the experience by saying someone has "passed" or "passed on." The truth is they *died*. But, saying someone has "passed" sounds less abrupt, less painful and is, therefore, appropriate.

Unfortunately, many of us have abused the value of political correctness in terms of how we communicate *to ourselves*. Political correctness is something we use and should use when referring *to others*. However, when we use politically correct terms to describe ourselves, we cause ourselves harm.

I took you through the mirror exercise earlier in order to illustrate that unless you're in a fun house, the mirror doesn't lie. We do. *We lie*. But we don't lie overtly. Most of us don't say things like, "I'm in the best possible shape of my life." Instead we use what I call *language lies*. Language lies are negative, inappropriate forms of political correctness we use to *hide* the truth from ourselves. Language lies are words we choose to use when describing to ourselves what doesn't honestly or accurately depict our circumstances *in relation to* our desired goals. The intent of a language lie is to *deceive ourselves* – to keep us from feeling pain. The difference between political correctness and language lies is that language lies are used to dishonestly describe *ourselves*, whereas, political correctness is used to politely describe *others*.

Language lies keep us from seeing the truth, and they prevent us from reaching our highest level of health. Language lies are a defense mechanism that may protect us from physical and emotional pain in the short run, but ultimately imprison us and cause us tremendous pain in the long run. It is through the use of language lies that we rationalize why we look and feel the way we do – why our health isn't what it could or should be.

Whether or not language lies cause harm depends upon you. It depends upon what you want. If you want to change something negative in your life, then language lies are harmful. For example, if I were fat but chose to think myself merely "a bit overweight," yet I had a strong desire to lose weight, then thinking of myself as merely "a bit overweight" would be a harmful language lie. However, if I were to think of myself as "a bit overweight" and *didn't* really have a strong desire to lose weight, then this would not be a language lie. The difference between these two identical phrases – "a bit overweight" – is how they *relate* to my desired goals.

Despite its wonderful potentialities, for most people, the human brain really only understands basic signals of pain and pleasure. Use of the phrase, "a bit overweight" doesn't cause very much pain. *If it doesn't cause me pain, then my brain doesn't know that something needs to change.* In this scenario, my desire to lose weight and the language I chose to describe myself are inconsistent with each other, and therefore incapable of producing the desired result of losing weight. The inconsistency between my desired

The Honesty Diet

goal and the language I used to describe myself is a form of *deception*. Using the language lie keeps me from having to change – in this case, to lose weight.

Learning to recognize our use of language lies requires *honesty*. If our intent is to deceive, then we are using a language lie. If you're being honest, saying you are "overweight" is a less harsh word for the truth that you are *fat*. If you say you're fat, then you're telling your brain being fat is painful. Your brain will then start working on ways to get out of pain, or in this case, to lose weight. If you really want to lose weight but insist on describing yourself or thinking of yourself as merely "overweight," you don't motivate your brain to take action.

I once had a patient say to me, "You know, overall, I think I'm pretty healthy." I couldn't believe the degree of dishonesty this man was expressing. Only in his mid 50s, this patient was overweight, had high blood pressure, high cholesterol, and cataracts. He also drank a lot, slept poorly, had a high-stress career, barely exercised, and ate way too much trans-fat and other processed food. In addition, he took numerous pharmaceutical drugs on a daily basis to address the aforementioned problems. Lastly, he had an aggressive prostate cancer. If this is his definition of healthy, I can't possibly imagine what his definition of *unhealthy* would be! I didn't have the heart to tell him, "No, sir, you're not pretty healthy overall; you're just not dead yet. Somehow, you're still breathing."

All language lies we tell ourselves serve a purpose – they have a function. The purpose of this patient's language lie is to keep him from having to change his habits or lifestyle. By choosing to describe himself as "overall, pretty healthy," he is telling his brain that nothing needs to be done – nothing needs to change. Unless we are honest with ourselves, our circumstances and predicaments simply cannot improve.

Sometimes we completely absolve ourselves of responsibility for our dismal physical shape and health by blaming it on the largely misunderstood term genetics. People frequently say, "It's not my fault! My whole family is overweight. It's genetic!" Of course, this is a complete falsehood, but we'll address that subject more thoroughly in a later chapter.

Practicing Honesty

Let's practice being honest for a minute. Having done the mirror test on yourself, let's say you honestly saw yourself as either somewhat or significantly "overweight." And, in the spirit of *honesty*, what I really mean is the more honest description – *fat*. If you have acknowledged you're fat – congratulations! If you are fat, say to yourself, "I'm fat." Don't say, "I'm a bit overweight" or "I've gained a few extra pounds." Be honest. Tell the truth. Look in the mirror and say, "I'm fat." Being honest will instruct your brain to begin to correct the problem.

Stephen Covey, author of *The 7 Habits of Highly Effective People* and many other great books, frequently states "It's only the unsatisfied need that motivates." If you say you are a bit overweight or you could lose a couple of pounds, that doesn't motivate your brain to admit something

The Honesty Diet

needs to change. After all, if most everyone else around you is "overweight," why should you then change? You're just like everyone else.

Let's do another exercise. What is the opposite of "fat?" "Skinny," right? OK, what then is the opposite of "overweight?" Obviously, if we are being honest, the answer is "underweight." But how often do you describe someone as underweight? You don't. If someone is underweight we often say they are skinny. We wouldn't describe someone who is underweight as thin or slim because those terms would be more appropriate for someone who is neither overweight nor underweight.

Virtually the only time we use the term underweight is if we are referring to competitive boxers or wrestlers. So if we almost never use the word "underweight" to describe someone who is skinny, why is it we use the term "overweight" to describe someone who is fat? The answer is because the term overweight is a polite term we use so as not to offend the fat person to whom we are referring. Sometimes the term overweight is even too offensive, so we use even more creative terms like "big-boned," "curvy," and "husky" to describe someone. However, if we refer to *ourselves* as overweight, big-boned, curvy, or husky instead of what we really are, which is fat, then we deceive ourselves and perpetuate the problem.

Saying you are "overweight" is as dishonest as describing a poor person as "under-financed." Language lies soften the pain associated with being fat and, in the long run, exacerbate the obesity epidemic our country is currently suffering from.

Blinded by Language Lies

While vacationing in Florida I came across a fascinating story in the local paper. It was titled, "Obese less likely to view themselves as fat." The article described a recent study demonstrating that most obese people have a "psychological blind spot" that prevents them from recognizing themselves as obese. The study found only 15% of clinically-obese people identify themselves as obese. The researchers used the politically correct term "psychological blind spot" to politely describe these individuals. The truth is these obese people didn't have a "blind spot," they were just being *dishonest*. Eighty-five percent of these obese people were being *dishonest* with themselves. This same study also found 71% of normal-weight people classified themselves as normal weight.

To me, this study clearly demonstrates an inverse honesty-to-obesity relationship. That is, in general, the more overweight someone is, the more *dishonest* they tend to become about their weight. I was pleasantly surprised to see the researchers state, "such a lack of self-awareness can be deadly." Considering obesity has been credited as a leading cause of death in the United States, this was an important acknowledgment.

Another example of how using language lies keep us unhealthy would include the increasingly common, and dare I say popular, phenomenon of Attention Deficit Disorder or Attention Deficit Hyperactivity Disorder. ADD and ADHD are not new diseases. More accurately, they are not even *diseases*. Before 1980, ADD/ADHD had another name – a more *honest* name. Before the language lie term "ADD/ADHD" was *invented*, the formal diagnostic text for psychological/mental disorders (DSM-III-R) termed the condition MBD or *minimal brain damage*. The political correctness movement has changed this term to the much less painful, and therefore, much more socially acceptable ADD/ADHD. The problem with this language lie is that it *masks* the problem.

If your child is minimally brain damaged, you are much more motivated to try to properly address the problem than if your child just has ADD/ADHD. Besides, what motivation is there to help your child if he or she is just like every other one in five American boys who allegedly have ADD/ADHD? Changing the name of minimal brain damage to ADD/ADHD and pumping a child full of drugs is a *dishonest* way of *pretending* to address the issue. *Think* about it. Is the reason why a child has Attention Deficit Disorder because there isn't enough ADD medication in his or her body?

Language Lies and the Marketplace

Language lies permeate society on all levels. The marketplace is no exception. Clothes for overweight people are cleverly titled "plus" sizes. What does that mean? Your size "plus" all your extra fat? Recently, I saw them described as "extended" sizes. What the heck is an "extended" size? Is it for people whose bellies or butts "extend" beyond their reasonable proportions? Language lies are everywhere. A nationwide grocery store where I used to frequently shop has titled a small section in the rear of the store the "Living Well" section. What does this

Don't Take Advice From Fat Doctors!

imply? That the other remaining sections of the store are the "Living Like Crap" sections?

At the time of this writing, trying to prevent osteoporosis with calcium is very *en vogue*. People, particularly women, are being told the reason they're developing osteoporosis more rapidly than previous generations is because they aren't consuming enough calcium. Now, without exploring the validity of such an assertion (I think it is nonsense – American women consume more calcium than any other women on the planet!), let's explore the level of *honesty* of how some people attempt to address this problem.

There are people I know who eat calcium-enriched chocolates all day long. These chocolates are synthetically laced with calcium and vitamin D. Each bite contains 500 mg of calcium. Never mind the human body is thought to be capable of only absorbing so much calcium per unit of time, the remainder of which is excreted. However, these people don't just pop one or two a day. Instead, they eat three or four of these *candies* (that's really what they are) every hour! Yet, they tell themselves it is healthy to eat these chocolates all day long, especially when they can lie to themselves that they're helping to prevent osteoporosis. How *honest* is this? Do you really think you're going to be healthy eating chocolates all day? Do you really think the reason you're at risk for osteoporosis is because you aren't eating enough chocolate?

Fruits and vegetables also contain calcium that doesn't need to be synthetically added to a nutritionless substance like chocolate. But which one do you think is healthier, eating chocolate or eating fruits and vegetables? Now, I hear there are new chocolates that are "clinically proven" to lower cholesterol levels. I wonder if they have also "clinically proven" that these chocolates simultaneously cause cottage cheese on your thighs and acne on your face? Interestingly enough, one person I know who eats these anti-osteoporosis candies has gained a substantial amount of weight recently. Coincidence?

Similarly, our society in the last decade or so has been successfully swindled by the candy industry. Have you noticed? Abracadabra! What used to be called "candy bars" suddenly are called "*energy* bars" or "*power* bars"! The words "energy" and "power" sound much more healthy than the word "candy," don't they? Well, sorry to rain on your parade, but adding some protein to a candy bar doesn't make candy any healthier, just as adding vitamin C to bullets doesn't make bullets any less deadly (punch line credit to Jay Leno)! Yet, I know lots of people who go around eating the so-called "energy" bars, telling themselves that what they're eating is healthy. But no matter what the wrapper looks like, and no matter how the manufacturer claims to enhance it, it is still candy! So ask yourself, do you think the reason you aren't healthy and fit is because you aren't eating enough candy bars?

~ 9 ~

CHOICE, DECISION & ACTION

Up until this point, I have used the terms *choice* and *decision* interchangeably. While choice and decision are frequently synonyms, they, in fact, are not the same things, especially in the context of health. However, let's discuss choice and decision in a context *outside* of health so we can truly embrace the concept and the distinction *before* applying them to our health.

A *choice* is an opportunity to select between two or more things, or an opportunity to act or to not act upon something. A *decision*, on the other hand, is a commitment, often an irrevocable one. Just semantics? Perhaps. However, wars are fought and people kill each other over semantics. So, contrary to what most people think, semantics are *very* important.

A choice *isn't* a decision. A choice *becomes* a decision. A choice becomes a decision only when acted upon or when a deadline has passed. So, the difference between a

The Honesty Diet

choice and a decision is the occurrence of an *action*, or the passage of *time*. Choice exists *until* action is taken with regard to any particular choice. Although it has become common in everyday language, we don't *make* choices... we *have* choices. We *have* choices and we *make* decisions.

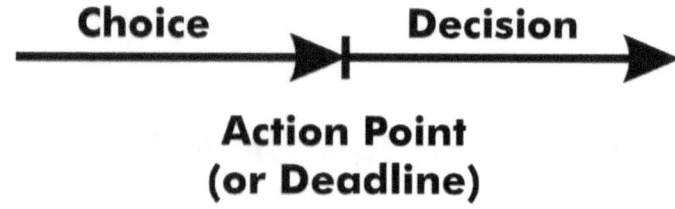

**Action Point
(or Deadline)**

Decision also involves qualities that choice does not, such as responsibility and accountability. Choice doesn't necessarily involve either of these, at least not until acted upon. Decision inherently possesses a quality of firmness and finality – of importance and consequence. In common usage, choice implies a more lighthearted quality of preference without consequence. Decision, on the other hand, possesses a more heavy-hearted quality of responsible accountability for any consequences of such a decision.

Which is Stronger? Choice or Decision?

On the surface, decision appears to be stronger than choice. A perception exists that *choice* applies to less important tasks. You could *choose* the color of your car, for example. However, an army general would not choose to send his troops into battle. He would *decide* to. Decision involves recognition of authority, either yours or someone else's. If a father were to select which college his child would attend, do you think he would say, "I have *chosen* that you will go to X University." Or, do you think he would say, "I have *decided* you will go to X University?"

However, I believe *choice* is just as strong as decision. At times, choice can even be stronger than decision. Decision only *appears* stronger because of its irrevocable quality – its sense of permanence. However, such a quality is not always a sign of strength, but at times, can also be a sign of weakness, fear, rigidity, even imprisonment. Decision only appears stronger than choice *relative* to the current level of awareness. Decision drives us forward in life – the decision to leave home, the decision become a professional or start a business, the decision to marry or divorce, the decision to have children, the decision to buy a home, the decision to retire. Decision sets us off on a course of action – a course of action many choose to believe is irrevocable.

Like many things, decision is a double-edged sword. Decision creates focus, and it can be a very powerful tool when a decision is made that serves us. However, decision can be an equally destructive tool when a decision is made that does not serve us. When a person *decides* to lose weight, to eat only organic foods, or to no longer smoke, that person has most likely made a decision that will serve them. When a person mentally *decides* they will always be fat, will never be out of pain, or will probably not beat cancer, that person has made a decision that most likely will harm him or her. Whether or not a decision serves us

The Honesty Diet

is a matter of inward honesty and can only be determined by the individual making the decision.

The Balance Between Choice and Decision

Decision is a commitment. By definition, it suggests rigidity. Choice, on the other hand, is an option. It implies flexibility and freedom. Both decision and the *perception* of choice are required in the progression, maintenance, and/or restoration of health. Therefore, choice, decision, and awareness have a powerful relationship to one another. That relationship can be expressed as the Chinese symbols yin and yang – where choice represents yin, and decision represents yang. In between the two is awareness – the liaison or gateway between choice and decision.

The Decision / Choice Relationship

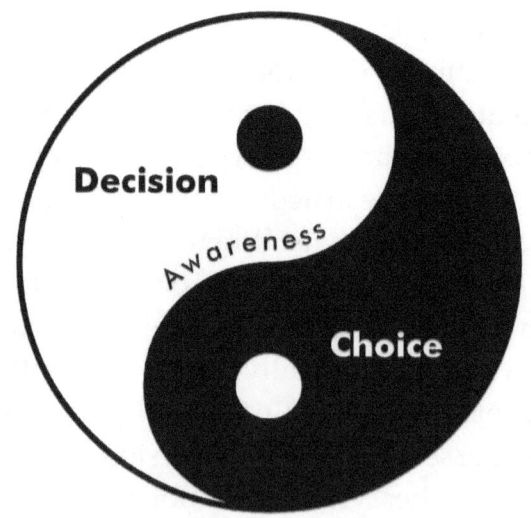

The Cycle of Choice

In life we are presented with choices. At many points we make decisions which take our lives in specific directions. Frequently, we believe these decisions remove choice from our lives. However, all we must do to once again possess choice is to raise our awareness. As we have already discussed, higher levels of awareness are achieved through the constant merging of honesty and education. When we successfully raise our awareness, we then discover that we once again have choice. The more often we raise our awareness, the more choice we produce in our lives. The more choices we recognize we have, the healthier we can become. The cycle continues endlessly. Furthermore, your quantity and quality of choice increases as a function of your level of awareness.

As awareness increases, choice increases.

For example, let's say you are on a treasure hunt in an imaginary underground maze. You come to a point where there are three tunnels to choose from. You have three choices and must *make* one decision. Once you *decide* on which tunnel to take, the entrance closes behind you. You cannot go back. You seem to have lost your freedom. Now, if you give up and believe you have no more options, then you're finished. You're going to be trapped in the tunnel. However, if you choose to continue down the tunnel you will eventually become aware that there are even more tunnels to *choose* from, and once again, you have another decision to make. This illustrates the point

The Honesty Diet

of the perpetual cycle of choice. We *always* have choice. Even after we *decide* on a course of action, we still have choice, although a *different* set of choices may present themselves. People tend to make decisions they *believe* set them on an irrevocable course. Sometimes these decisions have to do with relationships, sometimes they have to do with career, and frequently they have to do with health.

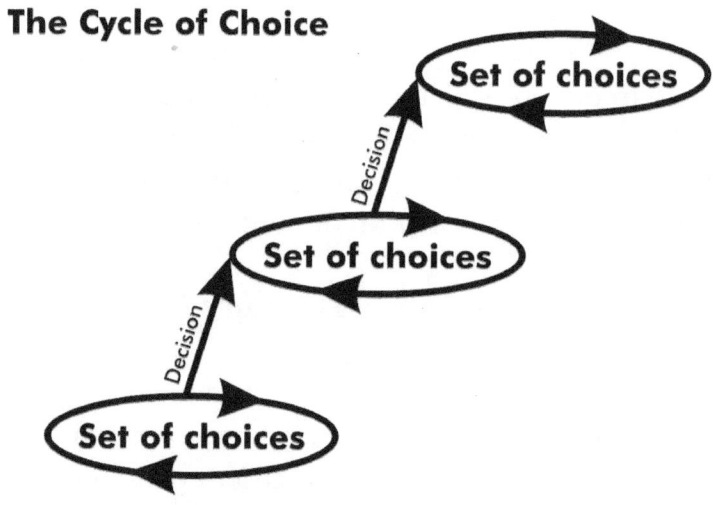

The Cycle of Choice

For example, an overweight woman might say, "I am overweight, because I had three children!" In her mind she has *decided* having children wrecks a woman's body and has caused her to be overweight. At any time she could choose to recognize this belief, this decision (or this decision to believe such) isn't true. There are millions of examples of women who have had *at least* three children, and the experience didn't wreck their bodies. But to recognize this – and not just attribute the other women's success to genetics – would require a shift in consciousness, a raising of her awareness. If, through honesty and education, she would raise her awareness, she would quickly find herself with a new set of choices. Choices that might cause her to ask better questions of herself such as, "How can I get control of my body and lose weight even though I've had three children?" This would be a much healthier thought with the capacity to produce healthier *decisions* in this woman's life, and would undoubtedly yield healthier *results*.

When you find yourself off the cycle of choice, raise your awareness and get back on. Raising awareness is the remedy for bad decisions that no longer suit you. Higher awareness is a *product* of good decisions – decisions made through honesty and education.

How does all this relate to your health? How does someone still have choice if they have already decided they aren't healthy? The answer to that question is the same one that got us there in the first place – decide! *Decide* to raise your level of awareness. Your health is a product of the choices you *perceive* you have and the decisions you subsequently make – and your *perception* of choices is a function of your awareness.

With regard to health, short of most surgeries, virtually nothing is irrevocable. Therefore, choice still exists. The capacity to act, to choose, still exists. Being fat, being ill, and being lazy are not irrevocable decisions you have made. They are choices you have on a daily basis.

Choices you still have today, tomorrow and the next day. If you wish to become healthy, fit, or energetic you must recognize your choices and decide to become so each and every day. You don't just decide to be healthy, fit, or thin once last week or last month, you *decide* to be these things *daily*.

Giving up and saying something like, "I am just a fat person" is only a *decision* made in one's *present* awareness. I say *present* awareness because, honestly, there isn't any reason why a person couldn't still *choose* to not be fat, right now. When you decide something destructive like "I'm just a fat person" you *imprison* yourself and *eliminate* the perception of choice. You end the cycle of choice. People tend to think that once you make a decision, you are imprisoned by that decision because decision means "irrevocable." This is true, but *only* if you are unable to raise your awareness. When you do decide to raise your awareness, you again return to the cycle of choice. As we will thoroughly explore in a later chapter, blaming our poor health or disease on genetics is a *decision* of permanence, though a false one. The perception exists among most doctors and patients that genetics have been "decided" for us. Nothing could be farther from the truth.

"I Don't Have a Choice!"

One of the most common statements I hear is the highly dishonest phrase, "I don't have a choice!" which also demonstrates a real lack of awareness. We *always* have choice. But we just frequently *choose* not to recognize our choice. When you find yourself thinking you don't have a choice *that* is usually a good indication you are resisting change or are defending a personal rule that isn't serving you.

For example, let's say a man proclaims, "I don't have a choice. I have to work at that awful job. Otherwise I can't feed my family." Don't you feel sorry for his plight? How awful it must be to not be able to feed one's family. Well, is this really true? Does he really not have any choice? Why does he say that? Does he mean he couldn't find a job at another company or business? Why not? What is stopping him? Does someone have a gun to his head forcing him to go to work at that same job day after day?

Some of you may assume this situation might apply to a poorer person working at a low-paying job. However, the person I'm modeling this example after is someone I know. He is a highly paid middle manager for a Fortune 500 company. He has four children, a materialistic, high-maintenance spouse, an enormously expensive house, and four cars (one of which is a Ferrari). Yet, he adamantly suggests he doesn't have a choice. He insists he *has* to work at this job so he can feed his family. Do you still feel sorry for him? He's not being very honest with himself, is he? If he were to practice some inward-honesty and clarify his values, he may come to recognize that he arguably has more choice than millions of people in the United States have.

Your brain only follows directions. When you insist you "don't have a choice" your brain accepts your word as truth and simply stops working. Saying you do not have a choice is an excuse, a prison, a copout and just plain dishonest. Many people say they "don't have a choice," but what they really mean is, "I could make that decision, but then I'd have to change." Recognizing you have choices does not mean those choices are without consequences or discomfort. For example, "I'd like to live in New York City, but then I'd have to move to the East Coast." Well, duh! Of course you'd have to move to the East Coast. That's where New York is! So, "I don't have a choice" really is just an excuse for not *wanting* to change.

Not All Choices Are Conscious

It should be made clear when I use the words choice and decision I do not necessarily mean all choices and decisions are made *consciously*. In fact, in any given day I would argue human beings make more decisions subconsciously and unconsciously than we do consciously. However, most people think they make conscious decisions. One of the goals of this book is to bring to the surface many of these unconscious decisions we make each and every day, then convert them to conscious decisions and direct those decisions toward health instead of sickness, toward fitness instead of fatness.

The Power of Decision

In 49 BC, Julius Caesar marched his army toward Rome. He crossed a small river in northern Italy, called the Rubicon. It served as an informal border between the northern Roman provinces and Italy proper. Crossing the

Rubicon represented an irrevocable decision. Caesar's army would, indeed, attack Rome. At this time Caesar allegedly uttered the phrase, *"alea iacta est"* which meant, *the die is cast*. Therefore, "crossing the Rubicon" is a phrase that has come to mean any person making an irreversible decision – or passing the point of no return.

Fifteenth-century Spanish explorer Hernando Cortés is often associated with the extinction of the Aztec Empire. He is, perhaps, better known for setting fire to his own ships upon arriving in Mexico as a symbol of his irrevocable commitment to succeed and to completely eliminate any notion of retreat by either himself or his men.

These allegedly true stories of history are meant to illustrate the difference between *choice* and *decision*. The primary distinction being that decision precludes going back upon or altering a choice once made. Decisions guide our actions. Decisions *create* focus and clarity. Decisiveness is a quality identified by many famous business people as a required attribute for success.

The Weakness of Decision

Decision can also be a source of tremendous weakness. While decision creates focus and clarity, it simultaneously creates tunnel vision. Decision has a tendency to narrow your world because it creates rigidity, an inability to adapt to changing circumstances and environments. Decision functions a lot like blinders on a carriage horse. The blinders are meant to keep the horse *focused* on what is immediately in front of him and not be distracted by the things going on around him. Our objective, then, is to learn to balance decision and choice in proportion to one another.

For example, if you *decide* to lose weight and live a healthier lifestyle, you must be willing to recognize when your efforts do not support your decision. Let's say in your decision to lose weight, you find your weak knees make it difficult for you to jog. This doesn't mean you eliminate exercise from your weight-loss plan. Instead, you must be willing to take up an activity less strenuous on the knee joint to fulfill your decision. Perhaps an elliptical trainer or swimming would be a healthier choice.

Decision Means Action

Have you heard this story? "Five cats are sitting atop a fence. Two of them decide to jump off. How many are left? If you said "three," you'd be incorrect. The correct answer is still five. Deciding to jump off the fence isn't the same as actually jumping off the fence. Only when the two cats actually take action and jump off the fence will there be three cats left on the fence."

This is a story frequently told in personal development books and at motivational seminars. However, I think this story is flawed. These storytellers think *deciding* to do something and acting upon a decision are different things. They aren't. Decision is action. Decision means action. If you haven't *acted*, you haven't *decided*. If you haven't acted, then you still have a choice to decide or not to decide.

Decision without action isn't a decision.
It's still a choice.

> "To know and to act are one and the same."
>
> – Philosopher, Wan Yang Ming

The Meaning of "Decide"

The word "decide" is made up of two words. In Latin, "de" meaning *from*, and "caedere" meaning *to cut*. So "decide" literally means "to cut from" or "to cut off from." When you cut yourself off from something, you have taken decisive action. Therefore, instead of the arbitrary selection of something, decision is more the *exclusion* of all but one. So when you consider one of the premises of this book, raising your awareness, the notion of decision begins to take on more meaning.

Healthy people make healthy decisions.
Sick people make sick decisions.

That is, healthy people *cut themselves off from* things that make them sick, such as cigarettes, alcohol, sleepless nights, destructive friends, family and business partners, sedentary lifestyles, and gluttony. Conversely, sick people *cut themselves off from* things that make them healthy, such as eating properly, sleeping and exercising. So, when people ask for the secrets of becoming and staying fit and

The Honesty Diet

healthy they are often looking for things they need to *do*. In reality, it is often the things we *do not do* that make us healthy – for instance, not eating French fries and *not* drinking sodas.

Many personal development experts recognize our *decisions* determine our quality of life. If that is true, and if *decide* literally means "to cut off from," then it could be argued it is the things we *cut ourselves off from* (as opposed to the things we indulge in) that determine the quality of our lives. Is it possible, then, in order to succeed in any endeavor, all we need to do is cut ourselves off from those things *actually* preventing success? If so, what are those things that prevent success? I firmly contend the things preventing success in the areas of health, weight loss, or any other important area can be identified through *honesty*. Health, in many respects, is the favorable result of the things we cut ourselves off from.

The Prison of "How"

One of the most frequent questions I am asked is, "How? *How* do I change? *How* do I heal? *How* do I lose weight? *How* do I become more healthy?" The irony of *how,* is that although it makes it sound as if someone wants to change, often they really don't. They use *how* as an excuse – as an attempt to convince themselves they lack the ability or knowledge to change.

Change requires a shift, a shift of position, both physical and psychological. For example, in a televised interview with Larry King, Anthony Robbins once pointed out that in one study those who succeeded in their efforts

Don't Take Advice From Fat Doctors!

to quit smoking did so by simply *deciding* to quit. They simply changed their sense of identity from that of a smoker to that of a nonsmoker. Those who most struggle to quit smoking are those who still fundamentally "see" themselves as a smoker. Those who successfully quit smoking did so cold turkey. They merely *decided* one day, not that they do not smoke, but that they are no longer a smoker. Do you hear the difference? One is an activity; the other is an identity.

In the first scenario, the person still identifies himself or herself as a smoker who is *trying* to stop the *activity* of smoking. In the second scenario, the person no longer "sees," himself or herself, as a smoker. Since their identity is no longer that of a smoker, quitting isn't difficult for them. Those people shifted their consciousness – their identity – from that of a smoker to that of a non-smoker.

What "how" really means is "I don't *want* to change." Or, "I don't want to change, *yet*." Or, "I want to change *as long as I don't have to change anything!*" For example, I have a friend who is concerned about developing Alzheimer's disease and osteoporosis. Almost every time I see her she asks me how she can prevent these diseases from happening to her. After reminding her these diseases don't happen to us, we choose them daily, I then tell her numerous physical and mental strategies for preventing the development of these diseases. But she never implements them. The next time I see her, she asks me the same question, "How do I prevent these diseases?" The reason she asks me the same questions over and over again is not because she's already started to develop Alzheimer's, but because she doesn't really

The Honesty Diet

want to prevent those diseases. Or, perhaps I should say she isn't willing to alter her current lifestyle, and risk possibly becoming slightly uncomfortable in the process, to prevent the development of such diseases. Can you see how *how* is an excuse? It's a delay tactic. It's an attempt to convince yourself you are unable to change. When someone says, "How?" what that really means is they haven't *decided* to change yet.

Some people might think this *how* issue is off base. "But I really don't know how to make these changes," some people say. I firmly disagree. There is an *honest* use and a *dishonest* use of the word *how*. Not knowing how to do *everything* is not what I mean. For example, I do not know how to fly an airplane. However, if I *decided* I wanted to learn how to pilot, I would know what to do. For starters, I'd have to contact a flight school. This would be an honest use of the word "how."

Many people, however, dishonestly use the word how. They use it as an excuse for not changing or for not following through. For example, let's say you really wanted (*but had not yet decided*) to lose weight. Many people say they do not know *how* to lose weight. I would suggest this is nonsense. People who want to lose weight or stop smoking decide to lose weight or stop smoking. They do not say, "*How* do I lose weight? *How* do I stop smoking?" They simply *decide*, and then they do it. There is no issue, there is no obstacle. *The how is a product of decision*. Once you *decide*, the *how* presents itself.

Everybody, and I mean everybody, knows *how* to lose weight. However, most people do not *want* to lose weight. I'm serious. In order to lose weight permanently, you must be *honest*. But this is extremely difficult for most people. Most people are not willing to be honest with themselves, and that is why they don't lose weight.

People will often challenge me on this and say, "That is not true. I *desperately* want to lose weight." I then ask them, "If you really want to lose weight, why do you have diet soda in your refrigerator? Why do you have potato chips and cookies loaded with trans-fats in your pantry? Why do you eat late at night? Why don't you exercise daily? Why do you start off each day with a greasy egg sandwich from some hamburger chain and a chemical-laden doughnut from a coffee shop? Why do you buy high sugar "snacks" from the vending machines at work during the day? Are these examples of how you *desperately* want to lose weight? Seriously, do these really sound like *honest* efforts of someone wanting to lose weight and be healthy? Your actions and your words don't fit together. It doesn't really look to me like you have any real *desire* to lose weight and be healthy."

Obviously, the prison of *how* is not unique to losing weight. It holds true for just about anything. Just remember: if not used honestly, *how* is an excuse. It means you don't really *want* to change. Successful people rarely say *how*. They simply decide.

There's No Such Thing as Doubt

People who really *want* something don't have doubt about achieving that something. If you are feeling doubt about losing weight or becoming healthy, you must learn to recognize doubt is a secret code word, a language lie, if you will, for "I don't really *want* to change." This is something you will need to understand in order to move beyond your resistance and stagnation. Simply identifying and accepting use of the word "how" as a code for not really wanting to change, will catapult you half-way through your challenge.

Awareness Makes the Difference

One thing that has always intrigued me about people is how two different people can have the *exact same* experience, and yet come to completely different conclusions about that experience. For example, two people of equal levels of fitness (but not necessarily "in shape") go to the gym to work out. They both work out to the same level of intensity for the same amount of time. The next day they both have the same degree of muscle soreness. However, one of them says, "Wow! I can't believe how sore I am. I must have gotten a really good workout. I can't wait for the next one." The other person, who had the *exact same experience* says, "Wow! I can't believe how sore I am. I'm *never* going to work out again!"

I've witnessed this phenomenon on several occasions. Clearly, the reason there is such a drastic difference in interpretation of what the same experience means to each person is their *awareness* about what muscle soreness *means* and what they *choose* to associate the feeling of soreness with.

The first person chooses to associate *achievement* with muscle soreness. This person understands muscle soreness is a sign the muscles have been *successfully* worked out, and that they will heal and repair to become stronger and healthier than they were before. The second person chooses to associate *failure* with soreness. It hurts, which to him means he did something wrong, and he never wants to experience that pain again. How bizarre! If you had to choose between these two individuals, which would you more connect with? Which one most closely resembles your attitude and perception toward exercise? If you chose the second person, there is a good chance you're already out of shape or obese – if not presently, then you might be on your way.

~ 10 ~

VALUES

What Are Values?

Your health is largely determined by your values. The idea of values is one of my favorite topics to explore. Like honesty, values are another notion philosophers have devoted much time to. Some describe values as the standard or quality making something desirable. It has also been said our values guide our choices and behavior. Another popular contention is that values are developed early in life and can be quite resistant to change.

However, all of these descriptions are abstract and not very practical especially in a health context. When people think of values, they tend to think in broad terms. For example, they may identify values as freedom, security, significance and community. Although these may be true values for some, these rather generic, highly abstract words aren't always easy for all to relate to. For example, what is one to do with the awareness he or she values *significance*? So what? How does this help us, right now? What are we to do with such knowledge?

We need a practical means of identifying and evaluating our values. I've figured out an easy technique to help people identify their current values, evaluate those values, and decide whether or not to change those values. The technique is simple, yet extremely applicable and practical. Some may not think identifying one's values is an important element in losing weight or becoming healthy. However, I can personally tell you identifying your values makes achieving health goals much easier.

Value identification, or value clarification, is something not taught to most of us in school or at home. It certainly requires inward honesty, but it is also more than just identifying gut feelings, desires, or goals. Value clarification involves exploration of a level of consciousness most people reach only after they begin to embrace adulthood and the responsibilities associated with adulthood. Some people never consciously identify their values. They certainly have values, but they just aren't aware of them.

How does one identify one's health values, and how does one prioritize them? I contend you already know your health values on a subconscious level. In this chapter, I will give you techniques to extract your values from your subconscious, bring them to a conscious level, recognize them as values, and make them work to your advantage instead of your disadvantage.

The Honesty Diet

"It's Too Expensive!"

I have found that people can *always* afford that which they *value*. Expensive-ness isn't something determined by price, but by value. For example, when I was living in South Carolina, I noticed many people who lived in trailer parks somehow found the money or the means to possess valued items such as big screen televisions, cutting edge video game players, or flashy accessories for their classic, 1980s hotrod cars. Even if they lived in rundown mobile homes, they still found a way to own these "expensive" items. This is because they value entertainment-based items like big screen televisions and car accessories, and do not seem to value living in permanent, quality housing.

This is not a judgment, but it does demonstrate each of us can afford that which we value. Our values determine the decisions we make such as what to spend our money on.

Many people I have helped in the past said purchasing organic foods or paying for a gym membership is too expensive. However, when I ask whether or not they pay for cellular phones, cable or digital television, or high-speed Internet service they almost always say "yes." I also ask them if they spend more than $50 per month on beer and alcohol. I ask them if they own a digital portable music player, a digital TV recording system, a video game system, and a big screen TV. Sometimes these people answer "yes" to *all* these questions. I then ask them how they can afford these things. Aren't they too *expensive*? The reason they don't find all these things "too expensive" is because they *value* them. But when I suggest they start purchasing organic foods, they protest, saying it's "too expensive."

"No it's not," I say. "You just don't *value* your health as much as you do those other things."

My response has had a tendency to offend or make people uncomfortable. Uncomfortable, not because I said something offensive, but because they know they're *supposed to* value their health, but their decisions suggest the opposite. What they feel about *themselves* in relation to my statement is what offends – i.e. it is the truth that is offensive. Most people in the United States do not *value* their health. That is why so many Americans are sick and fat. It is why so many Americans feel they have to take prescription drugs – because they don't honestly *value* their health.

I easily spend well over $100 per month on various nutritional supplements. Some friends say, "Wow! That's really expensive." See? We have just identified that I value nutritional supplements, and some of my friends do not. To me, spending over $100 per month isn't expensive because I *value* the impact nutritional supplements have on my health. Others don't share this value.

"I Don't Have Time!"

Another version of the "It's too expensive" lie is the "I don't have time" lie, which is another means of identifying something you don't value. People always have time for things they *value*. For example, if you say, "I don't have time to exercise," that simply isn't true. What you mean is, "I don't value exercise." Or, it may mean you value

The Honesty Diet

other activities more than exercise. Remember: we *always* have time to do the things we value.

I always challenge people who say they don't have time to exercise. Invariably, these are the same people who go on and on about a half-dozen television shows they watch every week – representing six hours per week they could spend exercising. These people have the time to exercise, but choose to watch television instead of exercising. They don't value exercise as much as they value watching television. By the way, why couldn't they choose to watch those television shows while exercising?

We now have two simple and effective technologies for determining whether or not we value something.

> ***If you find yourself saying something is "too expensive," you have just identified something you do <u>not</u> value.***

> ***If you find yourself saying you "don't have time" for something, you have just identified something you do <u>not</u> value.***

These methods can help us determine what we do *not* value. However, what we are really interested in is a technology that helps us determine what we *do* value. That, too, is very easy to determine.

Identifying Your Values

When asked to identify or clarify our values, many people think it requires deep, intensive thought. We think it's something that can only be accomplished by going to a place of solitude, like the mountains or the ocean for several days and spend them pondering long and hard about what our values are. This is the romantic version of identifying values. Although it sounds very nice, this is not necessary.

Your subconscious knows all of your values, and believe it or not, they are right in front of you. Our job in the next few minutes is to reveal those values and bring them to the conscious level so we can be more honest, have more choices, and make better decisions in our lives.

Please take a few minutes and, on a blank sheet of paper, list all the things you *do* on a daily or almost daily basis. List everything you *do* consistently, and don't leave off seemingly trivial things, like brushing your teeth or combing your hair. Here is a sample list.

Wake up @ 7am
Take a shower, brush teeth, shave, and comb hair
Eat breakfast and feed kids
Say "Goodby" to spouse / say "I love you" to spouse
Drive to work, greet colleagues or an employer
Surf the internet at work
Eat lunch at a greasy, fast-food restaurant
Drive home, eat dinner, eat dessert, drink beer / booze
Watch the news on TV / Watch sitcoms on TV
Review finances, read a book, study a subject
Check calendar, make a to do list
Go to sleep at 10 pm or go to sleep at 2am

The Honesty Diet

Perhaps your list of things you do daily looks similar to this one. Perhaps it doesn't. Nonetheless, I would argue the list you have just made isn't simply a list of things you do daily, but is actually an accurate list of your current values. Could it really be this easy? Yes. This is the easiest and simplest way to determine your values. Let's look at this list more carefully.

- "Wake up early" – This may suggest you *value* personal productivity
- "Take a shower, brush teeth, shave, and comb hair" – These daily actions suggest you *value* personal appearance and good hygiene.
- "Waking up early, driving to work, and greeting colleagues" – These actions suggest you *value* "employment" or "career."
- "Surf the Internet at work" – This action may suggest you, in some way, *value* "shopping" or "entertainment" more than you do getting ahead in your career.
- "Watch the news on TV" – This may suggest you *value* staying current on world and local events.
- "Watch sitcoms on TV" – This may suggest you *value* "entertainment" more than keeping up on world or local events or exercising.
- "Review finances" – This may suggest you *value* financial security.

What You *Do* Is What You Value

Are you getting the idea? What you *do* on a daily basis *is* what you currently value. Values are not ambiguous. They are not hidden deep within us waiting to be discovered. Values are right in front of us all day long. Whatever you *do* is what you value. You can't say you value fitness, but only exercise once per week. If you don't exercise daily, or almost daily, then you do not value fitness. Similarly, if you eat like a pig, then you do not value fitness. Don't lie to yourself. Be honest. Accept that the things you *do* daily *are* your current values.

A friend of mine, for example, has a job in which he has to get up for at 2 a.m. almost daily. He finishes work, in most cases, by noon. He follows this schedule because he values having his afternoons free for competitive outdoor adventure racing. So, he values afternoon *freedom* and *adventure*, which may suggest he values deep, regenerative sleep less than other activities.

Go through your list of things you do daily and identify your values. When you finish you might experience many different feelings. You may feel good about the values you have identified, or you may not. You may even feel frustrated or a little depressed over what your current values seem to be. Don't worry. Shortly, we're going to discuss how to change your values if you didn't like what you discovered.

Don't Confuse Desires With Values

Desires are not the same thing as values. If, from the things you do on a daily basis, you experience boredom, anger, frustration, and resentment, then there is a good chance one or more of your *potential* values aren't being met. Write down what that feeling is. What does it represent to you? What's missing in your life? Is it adventure, security, or freedom? What are you longing for? Do you long to be thin, fit, or to be pain-free? Write it down exactly. Now, I don't mean to disappoint you, but what you just wrote isn't a *value*. If it were truly a value, you'd be acting upon it – you'd be *doing* it.

Desires are only *potential* values. The only way to transform a desire into a value is to act upon it. Much like the way choices become decisions *through action*, so, too, do desires become values.

Commitment Means Daily

Similar to what we discussed in our chapter on focus, how much you value something is determined by how *often* you do it, i.e. frequency. You value the things you do *daily* more than the things you do weekly, monthly or never. The more often you do something, the more you value it. If you are *committed* to something, you do it daily. For example, let's say you practice martial arts. Your classes are only held three times per week. You go to all three classes per week and rarely miss a class. Are you committed? I would say, maybe. Do you practice martial arts at home for at least a few minutes on the days when formal classes are not held? If you do, then you are committed. If you do not, then you are not committed. You may attend class regularly, but you are not committed. Therefore, martial arts isn't really one of your values. It's really more of a hobby contributing to another value you express daily, like exercise, entertainment, or stress reduction.

Changing Your Values

Can you guess how you go about changing your values? I bet you can. If you want to change some or all of your values you must *decide* daily to do *different things* than you are doing now. But in order to garner the *power* to *change* your values, you must first muster enough *honesty* to gain *control* and recognize the fact that it is you who has determined your values, and hence, your past and current position in life. You *must* take responsibility. If you're not willing to take responsibility for your current values, health, and position in life, you most likely won't be able to change.

Even if you can't accept the fact that it is your values that have produced the state of health you see in the mirror and experience, you must at least be *willing* to take responsibility for changing those values now. Nothing is going to magically change by itself.

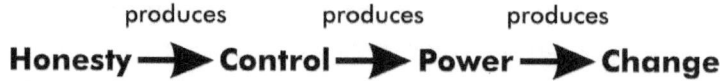

Responsibility vs. Fault

Even if your current circumstances are not your *fault*, you must decide now it is your *responsibility* to fix them. For example, it may not be my fault that someone burned down my house. However, it is my responsibility to remedy the situation as soon as possible. It is not the responsibility of the government, the fire department, or my neighbors to house my family and me. It is my *responsibility*, even though the fire wasn't my *fault*.

If you are fat, and are not willing to assign fault to yourself for becoming that way, you must at least take responsibility for fixing the situation now. However, if you do blame others for your present condition, you may want to reread the chapter on honesty and explore your "Yeah, buts." Changing your values, and therefore changing your life and/or your health, requires *control*. Whose fault something is isn't relevant. The only way to gain control is by taking responsibility.

~ 11 ~

IT'S WHAT'S ON THE *OUTSIDE* THAT COUNTS

> *"[Dad,] my teacher tells me real beauty is on the inside."*
> *"[No, son.] That's just something ugly people say."*
>
> – Actor, Jim Carey in "Liar, Liar"

When we were children many of us were told a language lie, which suggested physical appearance was not important – that it was what was on the *inside* of a person that counts. This is ridiculous. We may be spiritual beings, but we experience life largely in *physical* bodies with *physical* sensations and experiences. In fact, one way or another, nearly everything we experience in life has a *physical* component to it. Even emotions like love or anger produce physical manifestations in the form of substances like neuropeptides. These emotions further manifest in other physical ways, ranging from the words we choose for communication, to hand holding, to lovemaking. So, the notion we shouldn't assess or judge ourselves regarding how we *physically* present to ourselves and to the world at large is a *language lie* that has exacerbated the current U.S. obesity epidemic and our population's overall poor health.

When people say, "It's what's on the inside that counts," what they're often really saying is, "Please overlook my (or someone else's) appearance." We're asked to look to their personality, sense of humor, or good nature. We are asked to assess people based on their *internal* attributes, not their *external* attributes. We are supposed to weigh their *inside* qualities *more* than the *outside* qualities.

I disagree. Though it isn't politically correct to say so, this is really bad advice. Instead, I propose we should assess and evaluate inside and outside qualities *equally*.

I contend many of our personal qualities are often identifiable by our outward appearance. Of course, by outward appearance I don't mean whether or not someone is pretty or handsome. Beauty is in the eye of the beholder. I'm talking about the way a person presents himself or herself physically to the world. While you can't always assess someone's ethics, morals, or sense of humor from someone's physical appearance, you *can* get a feel for their sense of self-worth, esteem, and pride from their outward appearance. From someone's physical appearance you can often attain a sense of whether or not they *value* fitness, health, and/or physical activity. You can determine whether or not they *value* hygiene or courtesy toward others. You can get a feel for whether or not they might be lazy, unmotivated, or apathetic. Ironically, it *is* what's on the *outside* that counts. Or, perhaps more accurately, "What is on the *outside* is just as important as what is on the *inside*."

I believe this explains why so many couples tend to look similar to one another. I am convinced the reason a fit woman tends to be physically attracted to a fit man is because she can easily identify shared *values* with him like health and well-being. Similarly, unfit men tend to be attracted to and comfortable around unfit women because they also *appear* to share similar values.

I also think one of the biggest factors contributing to divorce in the United States is the change in *values* over time, which often manifest as physical attributes or actions. For example, when a man stops caring for his body, gains weight, and spends all his free time watching sports on television, that is often a good sign he's no longer very interested in spending quality time with his partner. Similarly, when one spouse begins spending a disproportionate amount of time working out at the gym, it is often because they no longer share the values of their spouse who might be at home stuffing his or her face with fast-food, alcohol, and chocolate cake.

So, while many think actions like infidelity are responsible for divorce, I would argue it is a change in *values* between a couple that leads one person to seek new companionship with another – perhaps someone who might share his or her new or existing values. This is not to condone infidelity. It's just an observation.

Attractiveness is a Product of Health

I've observed that people will do more for their *looks* than they will for their *health*. For example, people will try to lose weight more for aesthetic reasons than for health reasons. However, in reality, the best way to improve your looks is to improve your health. People actually do become better looking by becoming healthier. By the way, I've got news for you. All the makeup in the world, "slimming" black clothes, and loose, untucked shirts don't fool anyone. If you're fat, your gluttony is painfully obvious. Why not just become fit and healthy? It's so much easier!

Attractiveness is a *product* of health. As you become healthier your body will transform. Your skin and muscle tone will improve. Your figure will begin to define itself. Your eyes will become more brilliant and lively; the bags under them will diminish. You will emit a radiant quality others will take notice of and comment on. Your hair will grow, feel, and be healthier looking. The truth of the matter really is, you *do* wear your *inner* self on the *outside* of your body.

Am I suggesting health and attractiveness are the same things? No, but they do have one thing in common: body shape. While there may have been some brief eras in history where being a fat aristocrat or monarch was considered attractive, obesity was probably more a function of the perception of wealth. I sincerely doubt we will ever return to such a trend. In fact, in the United States (at the time of this writing) the opposite seems to be true.

Body shape can be a powerful measure of one's health. If you *value* health and take care of your body, you will have an attractive body shape. A physique you can be proud of. If you don't have a body you're proud of, it can only be due to neglect or dishonesty – and neglect is often a *product* of dishonesty.

Again, beauty is in the eye of the beholder. But, I think being unattractive is much more a function of one's lack of fitness, pride, self-esteem and self-control than one's genetics. I've seen what I consider to be the most attractive people become unattractive by letting themselves go physically. Conversely, I've also seen people, considered by some to be unattractive, transform themselves into striking, sexy people. They did this by raising their awareness – by deciding to value *self-respect* and *pride*, and by taking the subsequent actions needed to transform their bodies from a product of gluttony and neglect to one of attractiveness.

Several reality television shows focused on fitness have demonstrated this. As their bodies transform, the people on those shows exhibit tremendous increases not only in health and beauty, but also in self-esteem. Indeed, there is a strong relationship between your physical body and your inner feelings of self-worth. Unfortunately, the so-called "body-acceptance movement" has obscured and retarded this reality and accelerated poor health in America.

~ 12 ~

THE *BIG* LANGUAGE LIE

As we near The Honesty Point on our journey we come to a difficult pass. This pass – this awareness – can be emotionally challenging for many people. Indeed, this is the point at which many turn back. But I promise you, if you'll just push forth and continue, what awaits you on the other side will be well worth the effort.

When I discuss the notion of our wearing our *inner* values on the *outside* of our bodies, some would assert what I keep referring to is not "health" but "fitness." They then suggest that while they may not necessarily be *fit*, they are still *healthy*! This is what I call the *Big Language Lie* – the mother of all language lies and the epitome of dishonesty. It is this Big Language Lie far too many Americans use and abuse to avoid being honest with themselves about their health.

For the last 35 years or so, the public has chosen to perceive *health* and *fitness* as two different things – that somehow the two are separate or distinct from one another.

While there is a hint of truth to this, overwhelmingly the notion is dishonest nonsense. At some point over the last several decades, the political correctness movement (which would include the body-acceptance movement) began to distinguish between *health* and *fitness*. This distinction was not one for the better. Its intent was to *deceive*. The distinction suggested one could still be *healthy*, even if they were not *fit*. Interestingly enough, this societal distinction came into existence right around the same time Americans started putting on massive amounts of weight.

Many who read the early drafts of this book told me I had actually written two books: one on health and the other on weight loss. It was then I realized I, apparently, hadn't made my point, because this suggestion implies health and fitness are two different things. I adamantly disagree. There is, in fact, little difference between these two highly sought-after goals. It is this misunderstanding which accounts for much of the illness in the United States today.

Fitness and health are like two overlapping circles that *almost* perfectly line up with each other. The terms are overwhelmingly synonymous with one another. However, on very rare occasions, you could be *fit* but not *healthy*. For example, many of us remember Hall of Famer and Chicago Bears running back Walter Payton. By most people's standards, Walter Payton was *fit*. After all, he was a record-breaking professional football player. Walter died rather suddenly from a rare liver disease in 1999. So, apparently Walter was *fit*, but he was definitely not *healthy*. Many of us has probably known someone who was seemingly fit, maybe even slim, but dropped dead of a heart attack. Yes, it does happen, but statistically, it's pretty rare that someone who is *fit* is likely to be *unhealthy*. What is even *less* probable is that someone could be *healthy*, but not *fit*. It is nearly impossible to be *healthy* but *unfit*. Yet, this is commonly asserted by many Americans.

In 2003, an article in the *New England Journal of Medicine* rather definitively linked cancer to being fat. More and more scientific research is clearly demonstrating just how ridiculous the idea is that one could be healthy, but not fit. For example, being overweight (unfit) and having poor cholesterol health are nearly synonymous with one another. In women, being overweight and having imbalanced hormone levels also are often synonymous with one another. Both prostate cancer and breast cancer are specifically linked to being overweight. Heart disease, angina, and hypertension also largely coincide with being fat.

In 2004, the U.S. Department of Health & Human Services officially declared obesity a disease. Now, obviously, obesity is *not* a disease. In the overwhelming majority of cases, obesity is a learned condition – like bad manners or using foul language. However, I do think this erroneous labeling of obesity as a disease will inadvertently increase the public's awareness that *healthy* and *fit* are not different from one another. Why? Because if Americans think of obesity as a disease, then they can't simultaneously claim to be healthy, but fat. They can't honestly have it both ways.

Don't Take Advice From Fat Doctors!

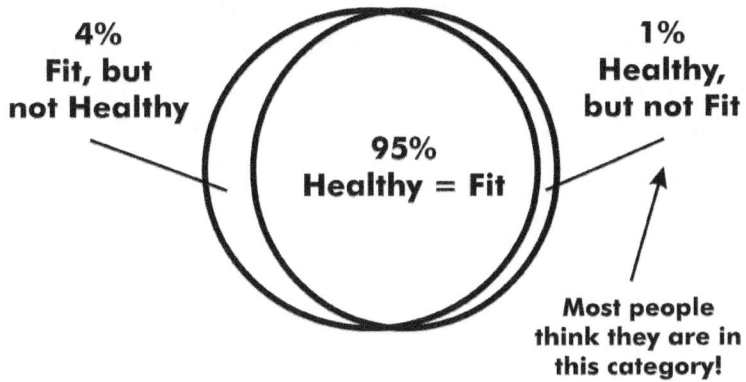

* This is a conceptual illustration, not a scientific illustration.

Let me summarize my assertion in the above illustration:

1. *Overwhelmingly*, you are healthy if you are fit – 95% of the time (e.g. modestly athletic)
2. *Occasionally*, you can be fit but not healthy – about 4% of the time (e.g. Walter Payton)
3. *Rarely*, you can be healthy but not fit – less than 1% of the time (e.g. an anomaly)

Interestingly, I would suggest most Americans place themselves in the third category of health and fitness, *even though it's virtually non-existent!* How incredibly dishonest! If you are going to take control of your health, then you must recognize that, in the overwhelming majority of cases, healthy and fit are the same things.

Healthy = Fit

The Honesty Diet

Therefore, the new awareness is that healthy means fit and fit means healthy. This does not mean that just because you're fit, you will not have any health problems or occasional challenges. Everyone has health issues from time to time. Perhaps, then, it would be beneficial to really nail down what healthy and fit mean.

Healthy or fit means:

- you eat a healthy diet (we'll define this later)
- you have an appropriate body fat percentage (typically less than 25% for men, less than 30% for women)
- you can easily do at least 20 minutes of intensive exercise (i.e. sweating) without dropping dead
- you do not have any adverse addictions, like smoking, drinking, or food bingeing
- you do not take <u>*any*</u> drugs (*Think* about it. If you were healthy, you wouldn't need drugs.); and, of course;
- all your body systems function correctly

This is not necessarily a comprehensive definition of healthy or fit. In fact, hopefully your definition of healthy and fit has a more rigorous standard. But any definition should *at least* include these parameters. Perhaps some doctors or health professionals might suggest this definition of healthy or fit isn't fair or reasonable. However, if you are being honest, anything less than these parameters, just isn't reasonable.

Healthy Means You Don't Need *Any* Drugs

Healthy means you don't need *any* drugs. This is another difficult awareness for many people to achieve. However, if you are being honest, this is strikingly obvious. In this country where we are bombarded daily in every media venue with the suggestion that drugs make us healthy and happy, people can be highly resistant to this new awareness. An inner conflict between what we *want* to believe and what our bodies know to be true can make this awareness difficult for people to acknowledge.

Because drugs often make us feel good, are usually easy to take, and rarely require changing our lifestyle, people often prefer taking drugs to the more *honest* acknowledgement that they are sick and need to make better decisions toward good health in their daily lives. It is their unwillingness to acknowledge they are actually sick that explains why they think they need drugs in the first place.

Now that we are starting to get into the *habit* of thinking again, let's *think* about drugs. Why do people need medicine or drugs in the first place? It's because they have a problem – something in the body isn't working properly. But when you take drugs, do they really *fix* the problem? And, before you answer, *think* carefully about what the question is asking. Does the drug *fix* the problem? Do you have to take the drug again, later? If so, was the problem *fixed*? Or, did it just seem to *go away for a while*? If your answer is the latter, then guess what? You're sick. Imagine having to take your vehicle back for repair every 12 to

24 hours. What would you say to the mechanic? You'd probably say: "Hey, you didn't fix the problem!"

I know it seems contradictory that if you need a drug to feel good, to function, to lose weight, or at least to lessen pain or discomfort, you are actually sick. It does *seem* contradictory because when we think of being healthy, we think of feeling good, functioning well, and not being in pain. Therefore we *associate* health with the drugs we take. But this simply isn't true. It must be recognized that drugs only attempt to *artificially* make us feel the way we are *supposed* to feel – the way we are designed to feel – if we aren't sick. I'm not telling you to stop taking drugs that have been prescribed to you. I'm just asking you to be *honest* about your current health status and admit if you are taking *any* drugs, then you are sick, not healthy.

What is the benefit of assuming this new level of honesty? Well, for starters, if you tell yourself you are sick, your brain will start looking for ways to fix the sickness – because that's what the brain does. You're more likely to start trying to fix the problem with lifestyle changes. But, if you just go around lying to yourself, your brain won't do anything.

Let's look at a few examples. What about people who take antidepressants? Why do they need antidepressants? Obviously, it's because they are depressed. But does taking antidepressants fix the depression? Sure, as long as you keep taking the drug! Does that make sense to you? Does it *honestly* make sense that the reason why you are depressed is because there isn't enough antidepressant drug in your body? The reason drugs "work" in the human body is because they *artificially* mimic natural substances, substances we, in most cases, can consume as food and/or create on our own if we make healthy decisions. Sunshine, *real* food, exercise, and excellent sleep all contribute to the cascade of biochemical events that create the healthy, internal environment needed to do the same thing antidepressants drugs do (*This is not medical advice. Do not make any decisions about stopping antidepressant medication without first consulting with your prescribing physician*).

How about antacids? Have you seen the television commercial where a fat father is about to stuff his face with a giant, greasy burrito and his family looks on in horror at the realization that they know he'll have terrible heartburn afterward? The father then proudly pulls out an antacid drug and smiles at his family. He knows he won't experience heartburn because of the medication he took *before* he ate his burrito. His family is relieved.

What's wrong with this? What is the father missing? He isn't recognizing the fact that the indigestion he experiences is a *message* from his body that he shouldn't be eating the things he chooses to eat in the way he chooses to eat them. However, to him the indigestion is just a nuisance and shouldn't ever get between him and his massive burrito!

"So what," you say? "So what if I take a lot of drugs?" Here's what. Many people still are not aware that *properly* prescribed pharmaceutical drugs are a leading cause of *death* in the United States. I emphasized the word "properly" because when I share that statistic with people, they often contend this can only be because some people don't take their medications as prescribed. Not true. The statistic specifically documents deaths caused by properly prescribed medications, not accidental overdose. It has been documented that *properly* prescribed drugs contribute to more than 100,000 deaths per year in the United States.

If you decide to embrace this new awareness – that if you need drugs, then you are sick – you will soon find yourself with many more choices in life and an opportunity to *really* improve your health. Continue to deny this obvious awareness, and you will likely travel down the same road as those deadly health statistics.

I Don't Know Health Is, But I Sure as Hell Want It!

One of the ways best illustrating how infrequently people think about health is simply to ask, *"What is health?"* About 95% of the time people answer this question not by saying what health is, but instead by saying what health is not. I've asked hundreds of people this question. These are the most common answers I've gotten:

- Health is not feeling bad.
- Health is not being sick.
- Health is not feeling pain.
- Health is not having any diseases or other medical conditions.

Notice that none of these answers actually say what health is. They all say what health is *not*. Let's try looking at this differently. What if instead of asking what *health*

Don't Take Advice From Fat Doctors!

is, I asked, what *wealth* is? Could we answer this question the same way the health question was answered?

- Wealth is not being poor.
- Wealth is not being broke.
- Wealth is not being in debt.

These definitions of wealth are pretty silly, aren't they? Not being poor or broke doesn't mean you are wealthy, does it? Not being in debt doesn't mean you are wealthy either, does it? Well, then why do we think health means not being in pain, not being sick, or not having a disease? The point is health isn't simply the opposite of being sick. Just because you don't have pain or a disease doesn't mean you are healthy.

Have you ever heard people say, "I don't know what happened. Yesterday, I was as healthy as a horse. Now they tell me I have cancer." People often have trouble believing me when I tell them symptoms are often the *last* signs of poor health not the first. In order for symptoms to show up, usually you have to have been sick for quite some time. Does cancer just show up overnight? Of course, not. When people *act* surprised upon discovering they are sick I try to point out what they're doing. "Why do you think you're *acting* surprised?" I ask, somewhat rhetorically. "It's because you've been *lying* to yourself. That's what *acting* is – a form of lying or pretending." Dishonesty is a powerful cause of poor health.

Health is simply the *product* of good decisions. Healthy people make healthy decisions. Conversely, *sickness*, in the overwhelming majority of cases, is the cumulative product of sick decisions. Poor health is the *product* of poor decisions. I repeat: *poor health is the product of poor decisions*. That means if you are fat, sick, or in poor health, it is because *you* have made fat, sick, or poor decisions. It *is* your fault. It is *your* doing. And... this is a *good* thing! You *want* it to be your fault. You should be glad it's your fault because that means you have control! If you had control to make yourself fat, sick, or in pain, then you also have control to make yourself healthy and fit again through decision – the very same way you became fat and sick. No, "Yeah, buts," please. Embrace this awareness and *decide* to become healthy again.

Disease Is Not a "Thing"

Not only do people not know what health is, they also don't understand what disease is. Most people think disease is a *thing* waiting to pounce upon them. However, this is dead wrong. Disease is not a thing. A pencil is a thing. You can touch it. A plant is a thing. You can touch a plant. You can't touch a disease. You don't open up a medical diagnostic book and look at pictures of a disease. You can only look at the *effects* of disease. Disease is a *circumstance,* a set of conditions – it is not a thing.

I like to use the analogy of a traffic jam to explain what disease is, and like disease, a traffic jam is not a thing. You can't pick up or touch a traffic jam. Rather, a traffic jam is a set of conditions causing traffic to not flow smoothly. Do cars by themselves cause traffic jams? No. Backed up cars are the *effects* of a traffic jam. Any number of things can cause traffic jams. They can be caused by pedestrians, stalled vehicles obstructing traffic, malfunctioning traffic signals, contaminant spills in the road, construction, sporting events letting out, or any such combination. Any single one of these conditions may cause a traffic jam. Furthermore, it can be nearly impossible to tell the difference between a traffic jam caused by a traffic accident and one caused by a sporting event letting out (especially if you are stuck in the center of the traffic jam!).

The same holds true for disease. Various circumstances can cause the same disease. For example, any number of things can cause prostate and breast cancer. Conversely, the same circumstances can cause *different* diseases in different people, depending upon any number of factors. However, the biggest factor depends not on a person's genetics, as most doctors and patients erroneously assume, but upon their *decisions*.

For example, bacteria alone may not cause a disease, but bacteria combined with a poor diet and poor sleep might. Exposure to a chemical toxin may not cause cancer by itself, but the chemical exposure combined with a stressful home environment and never exercising might. A person may never be exposed to a cancerous toxin or a harmful virus, but as a result of low self-esteem and consistently poor health decisions made as a result of low esteem, that person may develop a life-threatening disease anyway. You see, it is the *circumstances* that cause disease, not the presence or absence of a given toxin, germ, or bug. And, fortunately for us, we have a lot of control over our circumstances – *if* we're willing to be honest.

The Honesty Diet

Don't Take Advice From Fat Doctors

I am always astonished when I see chubby doctors or overweight health gurus on television promoting their new book or giving health advice to the public. Why in the world would someone take health advice from a fat doctor? Seriously, am I missing something here? How dishonest is that? The fact that fat doctors write health books today is further evidence of our chronic state of cultural dishonesty. Think about it. If it were 30 years ago, and a fat doctor were to write a health book, he or she would be laughed out of business. Not today. Today, fat doctors who write health and weight-loss books are fairly common. Look around the bookstore. In the past twelve months I have seen no less than three health and diet books written by fat doctors and/or chubby health gurus! Only in the fattest, most dishonest country in the world could one possibly consider reading and following health and diet books written by fat doctors.

I recently watched a segment on a news magazine television show where a network affiliate was evaluated using a controversial diagnostic technology to see if 30 years of smoking cigarettes had produced lung cancer. He was quite fortunate. According to this new kind of technology, there was no evidence of lung cancer at this time. However, what was so incredibly humorous to me was this network affiliate was being read the results and lectured to about smoking by a fat, unhealthy-looking doctor! Where does the fat doctor get off lecturing this man on health? She's fat!

Don't Take Advice From Fat Doctors!

Several mornings per week, I watch a chubby doctor on a morning news show dispense health advice on a variety of topics. Recently, he was advising parents not to allow their children to drink more than four ounces of fruit juice per day, claiming doing so can contribute to childhood obesity. This health advice didn't seem to carry much "weight" coming from a chubby doctor (pun intended).

Years ago, I went on a Caribbean cruise. The cruise line offered free lectures on numerous subjects as part of the onboard entertainment. One such series caught my attention, "Live Longer and Feel Better." It was being offered by a doctor whose biography claimed she is "recognized as one of the leading authorities in the promotion of healthy lifestyles" and she "serves as the nutritional spokesperson" for a national organization. Sounds impressive, I thought. You can imagine my shock and disappointment when I arrived at the lecture to discover this "leading authority" in healthy lifestyles and a "nutritional spokesperson" was fat! To make matters worse, her advice was really bad. All I could think to myself was, "So if I take your advice, then I'll look as healthy and fit as you do? No, thanks."

If I were forced to take health advice from only one professional – either an in-shape personal fitness trainer or a fat doctor, without a moment's hesitation or an ounce of doubt, I would choose the personal fitness trainer – hands down. Why? Obviously, it is because the personal fitness trainer is more *likely* to be *healthy* than the fat doctor (*if* you embrace the awareness that fit means healthy). Personal trainers are more likely to be healthier than fat doctors, simply because they are fit! Many doctors work excessively long hours, consume massive amounts of caffeine, take excessive amounts of drugs and don't exercise. Sure, some personal fitness trainers may do this, too, but professionally they're less likely to do so.

There exists a perception in American society that doctors are smarter, more educated professionals than are fitness trainers. However, perhaps this perception needs to be reconsidered. As a doctor, I have come to recognize that doctors may have *more* education and *different* education than fitness professionals, but that does not mean that doctors have a *better* education than fitness professionals. More importantly, to *know* is not to *do*. Therefore, if a doctor *knows* how important being physically fit is, but isn't physically fit herself, then can she really *know* much about health at all? If doctors don't look healthy, then they don't value health. If they don't value *their* health, why would they value *yours*?

Perhaps it is worth considering that, in general, fitness professionals are *smarter* than doctors – at least with regard to the attainment and maintenance of *health*. Now, if we are talking about emergency, traumatic care, obviously, emergency physicians would be superior to fitness professionals. But this is a book about health, not emergency medicine, not disease treatment. Also, to be fair, I did once come across a business brochure promoting a fat personal trainer. Now that was laughable!

I think people are tired of taking health advice from overweight, over-stressed, over-medicated doctors. The era of "do as I say and not as I do" is over. We should not take health advice from fat doctors, and we should

Don't Take Advice From Fat Doctors!

not take health advice from nurses who smoke. *Have you ever noticed how many nurses smoke?* We all know this intuitively. However, for some reason some of us are still awestruck and mentally incapacitated by the sight of culturally-conditioned icons like a white coat and stethoscope.

I feel so strongly about this that I don't think it would be a bad idea to require all practicing doctors to be *physically* fit in order to continue to practice. After all, most states require doctors be *mentally* fit in order to practice. Why shouldn't *physical* fitness be deemed just as important? Fitness could be made part of their annual continuing education requirements. If they want to keep their licenses, they must have a body fat percentage less than 25% and 30% for male and female doctors, respectively.

Furthermore, if they wish to continue to practice, they should not be taking prescription drugs of any kind. Think about it: if they are taking high blood pressure medication, they certainly shouldn't be advising patients on high blood pressure, should they? If they are taking antidepressants, then they certainly shouldn't be seeing patients at all. Doesn't this seem more honest? Think about it. How would you feel to discover your airline pilot was taking anti-depressant or anti-psychotic medication?

My Personal Experience

As I have already mentioned, I wrote this book while I was virtually immobilized. I herniated my L3-L5 spinal discs while lifting weights (So perhaps you should not take any weight lifting advice from me!). At one point, the injury completely kept me from standing, walking, or sitting at all for several weeks. After that, for several more weeks, I could only get around the house with a use of a walker.

Unable to function without severe pain for almost a full year, I could barely exercise. It is well documented that just a few weeks without cardiovascular exercise can cause tremendous loss of muscle mass and cardiovascular capacity. That is exactly what happened to me. Although I did my best to eat as healthy as possible and get as much sleep as possible during those months, I never kidded myself into thinking I was *healthy*. Since I couldn't move my body, I couldn't possibly be healthy. My muscles atrophied, my body fat increased slightly, and I lost nearly all of my cardiovascular "wind." I knew I would get it back, but I didn't kid myself that I was healthy during that period of time. I wasn't. Because I wasn't fit, I couldn't be healthy. Period.

The Reluctant Awareness

I know the previous awareness – *that healthy means fit* – may be challenging for many readers. I'm sure lots of "Yeah, buts" came up, too. However, if we are going to become healthy and stay healthy there is another awareness that *must* be acknowledged – a truth we must embrace. This awareness is the logical and necessary conclusion of the Big Language Lie and it requires a level of honesty that few people in America today are comfortable recognizing. That awareness is as follows:

Fat = Sick

If you are fat – if you are overweight – then you are sick. Fat *means* sick. They *are* the same thing. You cannot be both overweight *and* healthy. Suggesting you are fat but healthy is an oxymoron. In the past few decades, new-age literature and some more progressive health and medical literature have rightly dedicated much discussion to the body and mind connection. This understanding has become so prevalent many have begun referring to it as a singular concept called the "body-mind." Similarly, if you can embrace this new awareness – that fat means sick – then we should start to refer to overweight Americans as "fat-sick" because, like the body-mind, these words are a singular phenomenon, *if we're being honest.*

One of our nation's biggest health problems is obesity. In 2004, the U.S. Centers for Disease Control (CDC) reported obesity was likely to surpass smoking as the *number one* cause of preventable death. The following year, an alleged "better" study adjusted that estimate down to the second leading cause of preventable death. Even though I read the follow-up study, it wouldn't surprise me at all to discover the statistic may have been "adjusted" down because we as a society were not *comfortable* with the conclusion of the first study and needed a more socially-palatable number. It seems we weren't ready for that level of *honesty*.

Now, of course, I can't prove this. I'm just speculating.

The Honesty Diet

Nonetheless, which number is correct isn't terribly important – whether obesity is the first, second, or seventh leading cause of preventable death in the United States. The fact of the matter is it shouldn't even be in the top fifty! It's an unfortunate statistical manifestation as a result of the lack of honesty we have about our health in this country.

Fat means sick. You are not likely to ever become healthy unless you can accept this new awareness. Upon acceptance of this awareness, you turn your brain on to solve the problem. The longer you deny this awareness, the longer you and your body will struggle for balance and for health. Can you imagine an alcoholic trying to become sober without first recognizing he's an alcoholic? Can you imagine a person in financial debt trying to get out without first recognizing she is in debt?

It is difficult to get people to accept this awareness because they must first recognize that *overweight* is just a language lie for *fat*. Then they must recognize *fat* means *sick*. Therefore, *overweight* means *sick* – something many people find too painful to accept. Nobody wants to think of themselves as sick, but lying about it and not recognizing it actually makes you *more* sick. The irony is if you'll just accept this, your brain will start to *solve* the problem. If you continue to refuse this notion your body will continue to become sick. This is especially difficult when discussing one's children. Pointing to a fat child and telling the parents their child is sick is painful for the parents. It's one thing for a parent to recognize they, themselves, are fat and therefore sick. It is another to acknowledge out loud and to others that your child is sick, because admitting this would also mean it is largely *your* fault. You're a bad parent.

When I was a youth, there was a cartoon on television that would often run safety segments where the show's heroes would teach their viewing audience something about safety. The slogan of the segment was always the same: "Now you know... and knowing is half the battle!" The same holds true for becoming healthy. You must know the truth. You must *recognize* the truth – and the truth is, *overweight means fat, and fat means sick*. Once you know this – once you recognize this – you are half way to solving the problem. If you don't recognize this, if instead you come up with a "Yeah, but," you'll probably never solve this problem.

Overweight = Fat = Sick

The Ever-Expanding Truth

As more and more Americans become fat-sick people's definition of "fat" seem to be shifting farther and farther away from reality. What used to be considered "fat" is now called "overweight," and what used to be called "normal weight" is now thought of as "skinny." Collectively, we keep *shifting* the definition of fat so as not to include the majority of ourselves in the definition!

I noticed this trend by watching reruns of television shows and movies during my back-injury recovery. One day, while surfing through the television channels, I came across a rerun of a 1990s sitcom starring a heavy, female comedienne. In the 1990s, this actress was considered by most people to be *very* fat, and for years was frequently mocked in tabloids and joked about on late night talk show monologues. She was without a doubt obese. However, when I compare reruns of this show from the 1990s to the people I see walking about today I realize so many more people today are the same size, often much bigger, than she was back then! By today's standards, many people wouldn't call the 1990s actress fat, but instead would label her merely overweight. I guess when everyone else around you gets fat, you look thinner by comparison!

However, does that mean most people today would perceive themselves as being overweight? No way. As we discussed earlier, a published study showed 85% of obese people did not identify themselves as obese when asked in an anonymous survey.

I also saw a more pronounced example of this by watching movies from the late 1970s and early 1980s starring actors like Chevy Chase and Goldie Hawn. Almost everyone in those movies is slim! I don't just mean the stars, I mean everybody. All of the extras in the movies were rail thin with rarely any sign of a fat person. And, if an overweight person did appear in the movie, that person today would, no doubt, be thought of as average weight! Use of this language lie has really gotten out of control. Instead of being honest and recognizing the truth, we continue to push back the definition of fat! It's by lying, using euphemisms like "overweight," "husky," and "big-boned," and it's by redefining "fat" that keep us from being healthy and fit, drive up health care costs, and lower everyone's quality of life.

Don't Take Advice From Fat Doctors!

Many years ago, I heard on the radio that the outdoor seating at Yankee Stadium in New York was being replaced. When the workers finished replacing the chairs, there were *several thousand less* than had existed before. The adjustment was made to accommodate the ever-increasing width of the average American's rear end. That's incredibly sad.

In order to achieve our health goals, we must first recognize and embrace The Big Language Lie: Overweight means fat, and fat means sick. Therefore, overweight means sick. Embrace this truth and watch your world (and your weight) begin to change. Reject this truth and you will continue to produce unsatisfactory results.

> *"According to a recent report, the average male waist size in the U.S. has increased four sizes in the last ten years, from 34 inches to 38 inches. See, here's my question. When are they going to stop calling it 'average'?" Just start calling it what it is... Fat ass!"*
>
> – Tonight Show Host, Jay Leno

~ Section Two ~

A New Perspective from The Honesty Point™

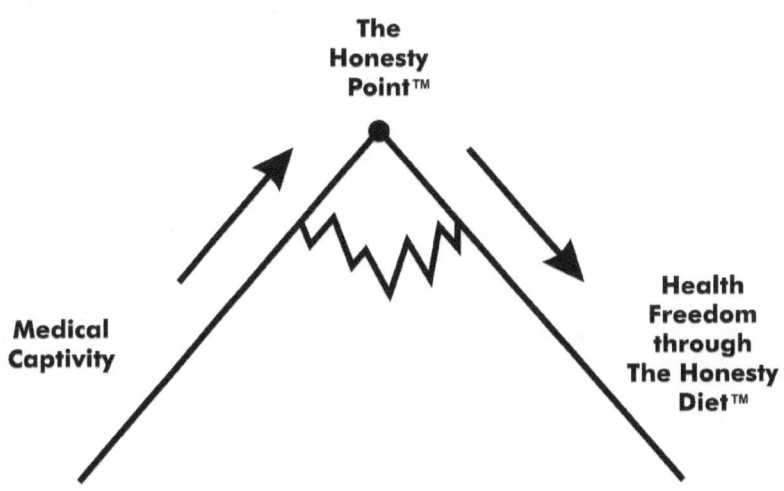

~ 13 ~

THE HONESTY POINT

Welcome to The Honesty Point. Congratulations! You've made it. Take a look around. It's really quite beautiful up here. The view from The Honesty Point offers a truly unique perspective shared by a few. If you haven't yet tossed this book into the fire, you are one of the select few. The view is unique in that it is, in fact, a holistic impression. The Honesty Point is the cumulative impression of all the aforementioned awarenesses discussed thus far.

    I may have insinuated that the goal of this book was to reach The Honesty Point. And, indeed, in many respects it is. For there is no Honesty *Diet* if one does not first reach The Honesty *Point*. However, as you can see, we are nowhere near the end of this book. We will spend some time up here on The Honesty Point, but from then on our journey will continue downhill. That is, with momentum. Reaching The Honesty Point is the prerequisite for understanding and embracing the Honesty Diet. With the momentum you have earned by reading this far and by thoroughly embracing each of the awarenesses we have discussed, you will find the rest of our journey easier on your feet and with the wind to your back.

Let's review the awarenesses forming The Honesty Point synergistically. We first recognized in order to get a different result than we have in the past, we must first be willing to *think differently* than we have in the past. We must be willing to let go of previously held beliefs that may not have served us. We learned to recognize we must genuinely express a *willingness* to learn new things and not just regurgitate beliefs programmed into us often since childhood without any evaluation or introspection.

We then reclaimed the capacity to think about our health by breaking free of *medical captivity*, a social façade we have been conditioned to recognize for the majority, if not all, of our lives. By first acknowledging the existence of medical captivity we were subsequently able to recognize this perceived dependency need not have any power over us and that *we can't spend our lives relying on doctors to maintain our health and still expect to stay healthy.* We embraced the idea that we, not doctors, not drugs, not insurance companies, are responsible for our health.

As we progressed toward The Honesty Point we came to appreciate the reality that it is our thoughts about health that produce the decisions we make about our health. It is these decisions and their simultaneous actions, nothing else, that produce the results we see, or don't see, in our lives. *The right thoughts produce the right decisions, which yield the right results.* Similarly, the wrong thoughts produce the wrong decisions, which yield the wrong results. These wrong results frequently manifest as obesity, chronic pain, diabetes, heart disease, and cancer. These common results are bad unless you don't mind them or *believe* them to be normal signs of aging – even if they are not.

We then visited the ingredients of the right thoughts, those qualities that produce the *healthy mental state* necessary for cultivating good health: focus, honesty, and awareness. We acknowledged that focus is really just a matter of combining *maximum clarity* of health goals (knowing exactly what you want) with *maximum frequency* (putting those goals in your consciousness on a daily basis). We embraced the idea that *commitment means daily*. You are only committed to something if you consciously acknowledge those health goals daily.

Our next stop along our journey to The Honesty Point was the exploration of *language lies* – the unique and clever words we use to deliberately deceive ourselves in order to avoid painful truths. It was within this exploration we discovered that *the primary cause of obesity, poor health, and most disease in the United States is the dishonesty we engage in with ourselves* on a daily basis. From there, we progressed to a simple, but powerful awareness that *healthy people make health decisions* and, conversely, *sick people make sick decisions*. This awareness explains why sick people have a tendency to become even sicker, not because they don't take the right or enough medications, but because they choose to continue to make increasingly sick decisions which, over time, worsen their health.

We acknowledged that, regardless of our present circumstances, we all have the power to change when we recognize we do, in fact, always have choice. Furthermore, we came to appreciate the subtle, yet powerful differences between choices and decisions. We identified the strengths and weaknesses of each and we accepted the notion that *a choice only becomes a decision when acted upon.*

We then learned how to identity our values and to differentiate between our desires and our values. We embraced the awareness that *what we do on a daily basis is a true representation of our values* and is indeed, self-evident in our actions. *If you don't do something, you don't value it, and vice versa.*

It was then some of us became uncomfortable as we discussed the societal taboo of outward physical appearance. We challenged and defeated the popular notion that it's what's on the inside of a person that counts, and not what was on the outside. However, after practicing our newly discovered honesty we came to realize *people do wear many of their personal values on the outside of their bodies* – their personal, outward appearance, if you will.

And, if that part of our journey wasn't difficult and challenging enough to our preprogrammed cultural beliefs about health, we then slaughtered another sacred cow. We recognized there is, in fact, little or *no distinction between being healthy and being fit.* We recognized this artificial, dishonest construct was the product of our society's collective defense mechanism established so we wouldn't feel bad or ashamed about the epidemic of obesity we have created ourselves. At the same time we came to appreciate if drugs truly made us healthy then people should no longer have to take drugs. We embraced the notion that a true, honest definition of health includes acknowledging *health means you don't take any drugs at all*.

Lastly, we put a final nail in the coffin of perhaps the greatest sacred cow in American society: the idea that you can be healthy, but not fit. Or, more succinctly, *fat means sick*. You cannot be healthy if you are overweight. It was then and only then we got our first glimpse outward from The Honesty Point.

The Honesty Point is the culmination of the all the previously discussed awarenesses. Yet, it is also much more than just the sum of its parts. As you embrace these new, honest awarenesses about health you will begin to recognize and appreciate a new perspective – a higher perspective. By embracing The Honesty Point you now have a much more accurate, honest, and acute perception of health than that of an average person. You now have the capacity for making great changes in your life if you so *decide*. The Honesty Point is the philosophical acknowledgement of an inexhaustible trove of *choices* available to you now that you have learned to break free from your medical captivity, recognize your values, and have begun to *think* again.

From now on, our journey will shift focus from reaching The Honesty Point and using the new perspective it affords to continue toward completion of The Honesty Diet. Now that we have explored the foundations of The Honesty Point and you have embraced the awarenesses presented within, we can begin to apply The Honesty Point in our practical, daily circumstances. But before we leave The Honesty Point and continue our journey downward, let's practice what we have learned by discussing three commonly misunderstood health topics: genetics, obesity, and addiction, and how these misunderstood topics relate to our daily health. Let's do so, not from an average person's perspective, but from the perspective of someone like yourself who has, with a considerable amount of effort, reached The Honesty Point.

~ 14 ~

THE MYTH OF GENETICS

Now, don't worry. I'm not about to suggest there is no such thing as genetics. Of course there is. However, I am going to argue an average person's current *perception* and *understanding* of genetics is grossly distorted and is hurting their health.

Why Fat-Sick People Like the Genetics Myth

Fat-sick people and much of the general public are attracted to the idea that genetics determines our health because the explanation is easy to understand and seems like a great excuse for living with and accepting their health problems. The belief is that something *outside* your control (your inherited genetics) is responsible for the current condition of your health and well-being. But in my opinion, genetics is just another way, albeit a quasi-scientific way of, once again, shunning responsibility and blaming our parents for who we've *chosen* to become.

Genes Must Be *Expressed* to Matter

As individuals, we may not have any control over what our genetic makeup initially is. However, it is becoming more and more apparent that it is the *decisions* we make throughout our lives that can significantly affect and alter the way in which genes are *expressed* or not expressed. Decisions we make can even affect *which* genes in particular are expressed and which are not. Merely having a gene means very little in and of itself. In order for a gene to be of consequence, it must be *expressed*.

The expression of a gene could be described much like turning on or off a light switch. When the switch is in the off position, the gene is dormant. When the light switch is turned on, the gene is activated – or *expressed*.

Many things within our control affect and determine whether or not a gene is expressed and two of the largest are 1) decision and 2) nutrition. And, of course, as has been previously explained, our decisions directly affect our nutrition. People are often surprised to discover that there is an emerging area of scientific study called nutrigenomics, which is the science of how nutrition effects the expression of genes. This field of study supports my contention that many factors, such as our food choices, largely determine the expression of our genetics – choices that can determine whether or not an individual will grow conditions like breast cancer, heart disease, or arthritis.

Don't Take Advice From Fat Doctors!

Of course, I must point out that I am not a geneticist. However, no matter how much minutia an expert may know about genetics, they may still fundamentally perceive the subject erroneously as a whole if the underlying assumptions behind their expertise are wrong. Sometimes, when you're too close to or too involved with a subject it's difficult to see the forest through the trees.

Genetics: The 21st Century Scapegoat

Genetics has become the lazy person's excuse for poor health. It has become America's ultimate, pseudo-scientific scapegoat. People in this country increasingly choose to believe it is not one's *decisions* that determine one's health, but one's genes. However, this harmful belief has one massive side effect: It lets people off the hook with regard to taking responsibility for their own health. No longer are people fat because they eat like a pig. They are fat because of their defective genes. No longer do people grow cancer because of their poor lifestyle. They "catch" cancer because of their faulty genes. No longer are poor cholesterol ratios a result of a poor diet and bad habits. Rather, genetics are at fault.

Because of this genetics myth people now believe their health is in someone else's hands – in something else's control. It is remarkably similar to, and perhaps just a variation of, the *medical captivity* concept discussed earlier. I am convinced that 20, 50 or 100 years from now, our present understanding of genetics will be mocked in a similar fashion to the way we now chuckle at how

The Honesty Diet

people used to think poor health was caused by evil spirits and demons.

Genetics Misunderstood

Ask one hundred people on the street what genetics is, and the results, no doubt, will demonstrate today's public perception of genetics is that one's genes determine one's health. Ask these same one hundred people two or three simple questions about what DNA is made of and how it works, and you'll find the overwhelming majority can't answer a single one of those questions correctly. Does it seem intelligent to you that the public has virtually no understanding of what genetics is, but is simultaneously convinced genetics determine one's health?

This phenomenon never ceases to amaze me – how quickly people come to accept as truth and gospel something they don't know the first thing about. It is amazing to me how quickly people have embraced the mysticism of genetics as the cause of so many health plights like obesity, heart disease, prostate cancer, breast cancer and even depression.

I suppose it really shouldn't surprise me, though. Blaming one's health woes on genetics is the ultimate "get out of jail free" card in the game of life. Can you imagine how liberating that notion is, how much responsibility is lifted off your shoulders when you *decide* to believe that genetics, not your decisions, determined your poor health? "It's not my fault. My whole family is fat…" "It's not my fault. My mother had depression..." "It's not my fault. Two of my relatives also had breast cancer." Believing genetics determines the quality of your health is basically a license to eat like a pig, not exercise and not take care of yourself. What would taking care of myself matter anyway if my genes are faulty?

Genetics has become the ultimate scapegoat – the ultimate excuse for poor health habits. And, it will be a difficult perception to break down.

"Genetics!" What Doctors Say When Stumped

Even doctors, who have had "more" education on genetics than the average person (but not necessarily "better" education), have fallen victim to the superstition of genetics. I have observed on countless occasions doctors simply blurt out the answer "Genetics!" to a question they obviously don't have an answer for. It seems saying the word "genetics" makes a doctor seem smarter than, perhaps, giving the more intellectually-honest answer, "I don't know." Personally, I'd rather go to a doctor who has the professional courage to say "I don't know," than a doctor who makes up answers they know may not be true because they fear looking inadequate.

Are Genetics *Randomly* Selected?

Will I lose my hair? Will I have bipolar disorder like my uncle? Will I be as tall as my father? There exists a perception that the genes you end up with are randomly selected. However, I contend that just because genes may *appear* randomly determined, doesn't mean they actually *are* randomly determined. I think within a few decades we will begin to recognize that genetics are not random. Just because scientists may not *yet* completely understand genetics' order, selection, determination and activation that doesn't mean they are necessarily random.

We humans have a bad tendency to assume if we can't figure something out, the problem must be unsolvable. Or, if we can't figure out an order, a pattern, or logic to something, it must therefore be random. We declare things to be random as opposed to the more honest statement which is, "At this time, something appears random. Thus far, we've been unable to determine any order, pattern, logic, or system to this phenomenon."

The philosophy of The Honesty Diet recognizes the parents' lifestyle and health choices, rather than their genetics, is a primary determinant of the genetics of a child. For example, a past acquaintance of mine has five children. Three of his children have what is described as a fatal hereditary disease which tends to shorten life to the mid-thirties. One of his children does not have the disease, and a another child is only a carrier for the disease. Seems random, doesn't it? I don't think so. It turns out that his oldest child does *not* have the disease. His second oldest child is only a *carrier* of the disease, and his three youngest all have the full-blown disease.

He and his wife, of course, have been told by their doctors this is just the luck of the draw – that there is no rhyme or reason why one child has the disease and another doesn't, that the condition occurred randomly as selected by genetics. I think this is unlikely. The fact that the first child was born healthy is a clue. The second child, only a carrier, is another clue. If you can put away any preconceived notion that genetics is randomly determined, you may notice that there is a progressive decline in genetic health from the first child to the last three. I sincerely doubt this is coincidence. Is it possible there is a reason for this seemingly random order of incidence of this genetic disease among these five children? I should also tell you that all five children are very close in age to one another.

Remember, people don't *have* babies, they *grow* babies. Babies are made out of the nutritional content of the parents, particularly the mother since babies *grow* for over nine months inside the mother. What do you think babies are made of? Where do you think they come from? Storks? Magic? Deities? They are made of the mother's nutritional content! If the mother's brain and body is made of junk food, then the baby's brain and body are made of junk food. If the mother's brain and body are made of healthy nutritious foods, then the baby's brain and body are made of nutritious foods. Isn't it reasonable to deduce that if a baby is *grown* in an unhealthy physical environment, that there is an increased likelihood that the baby may inherit and *express* genes for hereditary genetic diseases?

Bodybuilders know that in order to grow muscle several factors are necessary. Two of the most important factors are protein and sleep. If a bodybuilder does not get sufficient amounts of both, he or she can't grow optimal muscle. Which of the two is *more* important?

Successful bodybuilders will tell you protein and sleep are *equally* important. Successful bodybuilders understand muscle *growth* doesn't occur at the gym, it occurs in bed while sleeping. Muscle fiber *destruction* occurs in the gym. Muscle fiber *construction* and repair occur while asleep. Eight to ten hours per night of sleep is *critical* to a bodybuilder's success. If they don't get at least that much sleep, the body won't have the opportunity to re-grow the damaged muscle tissues. Simultaneously, if they don't consume enough protein they won't have the *materials* – the nutritional content – the body needs to re-grow muscle tissue. So they very much need both. Furthermore, bodybuilders can't work out the same muscle groups *too often*. Otherwise, they will retard their muscle growth development. Enough *time* must pass *between* workouts in order to maximize muscle growth.

Having children works very much the same way as building muscle. Having children *too often* or *too close* together and not adequately replenishing the materials – the nutritional content – of the mother *between* pregnancies can increase the likelihood of having children with hereditary genetic defects. It isn't all that complicated a concept to grasp. Growing a baby is hard work. It takes a tremendous amount of time and energy. Did you also know endurance athletes, like marathon runners, often develop respiratory infections within a few days of running a race? Why do you think that is? It's because they are *exhausted* and, therefore, have low immunity making them susceptible to illness. Do you think it is any different growing a baby?

Many people for lifestyle, career, or other reasons want to have all of their children within as short a period of time as possible. This may be a logical decision relative to their particular situation; however, it is a poor decision as far as genetics is concerned – as far as *growing* healthy babies are concerned. Women require a replenishing of nutrients between pregnancies, one of the most important of which is essential fatty acid replenishment.

Essential fatty acids, commonly known as omega-3s, 6s, and 9s, were historically found in wild, cold-water fish. However, today, due to pollution, they are probably safest consumed in high quality fish oil supplements. The proper balance of essential fatty acids is *critical* to a woman growing a healthy baby because essential fatty acids are one of the primary constituents of a baby's brain and body. Interestingly enough, the children with the hereditary disorder described above all suffer from a genetic disease in which essential fatty acid deficiency is implicated. Coincidence?

I contend that because this couple chose to have so many children over such a short period of time (due to religious influence, I'm afraid), it dramatically *increased* the likelihood of each child inheriting and expressing this recessive genetic predisposition for that particular disease.

This would explain why the couple's first child was born healthy – because the mother's body had sufficient levels of essential fatty acids and other nutritional content. The second child was a *carrier* of the gene, but did not *express* the gene because the mother's body was deficient, but not quite depleted of essential fatty acid content. However, by the time she became pregnant with her third, fourth, and fifth child, I suspect the mother's body was completely *exhausted* and *depleted of* sufficient essential fatty acids and many other nutrients required to grow healthy children without passing on their genetic predisposition for this disease. And yet, clearly, they were capable of having all healthy children since their first child was born healthy.

I would speculate that had this couple simply spread out their five children over a greater number of years, instead of cramming the birth of all five children into a much shorter period of time, there would have been greater likelihood of all five children being born healthy. However, lots of people have several children close to one another. Am I saying *everyone* who has children close together will have genetically defective children? No. Don't try to "Yeah, but" this. Don't try to escape this reality. Clearly, my acquaintance, his spouse, or both of them have a genetic *predisposition* for this particular genetic disorder. Most other people do not.

So I sincerely doubt genetics is randomly selected. It only *appears* random to people who have forfeited their innate capacity to *think*.

Genetic Health and Nutrition

We need to stop thinking in terms of ordinary "genetics" and start thinking in terms of "genetic health." That is, "genetics" are perceived to be fixed and "genetic health" is something we can affect. Your parents' nutrition and other health choices affected your own genetic makeup.

There's nothing you can do about that anymore. However, your nutrition and other health choices will affect what elements of your genetic makeup will be expressed. And, your nutrition and other health choices will affect what genetics you will pass on to your children.

We seem to have no problem understanding how smoking cigarettes before or during pregnancy decreases lung function in babies. We have no problem understanding how drinking alcohol while pregnant can cause fetal alcohol syndrome. We also have no problem understanding how smoking crack while pregnant causes babies to be born addicted to crack. But for some bizarre reason, we resist the idea that the food choices a mother makes before, during, and even after pregnancy (via breast milk) can increase or decrease the likelihood of growing a healthy baby.

Strangely, many pregnant women throw out all semblance of a healthy diet once they learn they are pregnant. It is almost as if they use being pregnant as an excuse to pig out and give in to unhealthy cravings. They will often, pretending to be half-joking, say frighteningly dishonest things like, "I'm eating for two now!" The implication being they need to eat *twice* as much food since there are now *two* people requiring nourishment. However, "I'm eating for two" is just a *language lie* people use to eat poorly while pregnant. Also, why would pregnancy suggest you should start eating poorly? Becoming pregnant should be an *incentive* to eat *more* healthfully, not an incentive to eat worse. "I'm eating for two now, so I'll have another apple" versus "I'm eating for two now, so I'll have another chocolate cupcake."

Sorry, but taking some prenatal vitamins doesn't make up for a bad diet.

The better the mother's diet during pregnancy, the higher the quality of genetics will be passed on to the child (in fact, the higher the IQ of the baby, too). The better the diet of the mother *and father* before pregnancy and the better the diet of the mother during pregnancy, the less likely a genetic defect will be passed on to a child. If you really think about it, this notion isn't much different from understanding the fetal alcohol syndrome phenomenon, yet we resist or ignore this simple connection because we don't like the truth.

Here's a good rule of thumb for selecting foods to optimize your genetic health:

If pregnant women shouldn't eat or drink something, then neither should you.

If young children shouldn't eat or drink something, then neither should you.

Always pretend you are pregnant and treat your body accordingly ...even if you are a man.

Genes *Follow*, Not Give Instructions

Genes are a lot like computers: they only do what they are told. Genes don't *give* instructions; they largely only *follow* instructions. The thoughts, beliefs and experiences we have and the subsequent decisions we make can impact the expression of various genetic propensities.

Earlier I described two people who went to the gym to work out together, but had completely different experiences. They had such different experiences because they both brought different thoughts, beliefs, and past experiences to their respective workouts. They also both brought different *values* and *motives* to the gym. Well, these same mental factors can affect the expression of genes differently, too.

Look at a set of genetically identical female twins. I like to cite examples using genetically identical twins because it not only helps illustrate how genetic predispositions can be expressed differently in two people with the exact same genetic makeup, but it also helps to illustrate how genes *follow* instructions instead of *giving* instructions. Additionally, published research involving tens of thousands of pairs of identical twins has shown non-genetic factors to be roughly twice as likely to account for common cancerous conditions as genetic factors.

Let's say the female twins have a genetic capacity to be tall. At birth they are separated and are raised by different families. An abusive family emotionally scars the first girl, while a benevolent family provides a nurturing environment to the second girl. It is plausible the first twin, due to chronic psychological abuse, may suppress the fullest expression of her genetic capacity to be tall. All other factors being equal, the second twin, the one raised in the nurturing home environment, is more likely to grow to her genetic height potential.

Phenomena similar to this fictitious example are well

documented. For example, children raised in divorced families or stressful home environments are much more likely to develop asthma and allergy problems than children raised in intact family environments. Here, the causative factor – the trigger of the genetic predisposition – is not merely the presence of a gene and an allergen, but whether or not their genetics were triggered – switched "on" – by an experience, such as, in this example, psychological stress.

It is also possible these same genetically-identical twins could have been raised in the same abusive household, but each *chose* to interpret and respond to the abuse differently from one another. While one twin may have been browbeaten into passivity, shyness, and fear – perhaps growing to less than her full genetic height or developing asthma– it is possible the other twin *chose* to block out or even defy the abuse, vowing never to let something like that happen when she raises a family and she perhaps, in turn, grows to her full genetic height or does not develop asthma.

What is the difference between these two identical twin girls in both of these two scenarios? How could two *genetically-identical* people have such different physical and psychological outcomes? I contend the difference between them is *choice*. Of course, these are only two, overly-simplified and theoretical outcomes of an endless number of possibilities. Keep in mind, I just as easily could have picked ovarian cysts, obesity and even cancerous conditions as the manifestation instead of a benign attribute like height.

Family History vs. Genetics

People frequently confuse family history with genetics, yet they're not *at all* the same things. Even many doctors seem to use these words interchangeably. To truly understand how genes do not imprison us and are not, in and of themselves, responsible for our health, a distinction must be made between these two terms.

In my family, there is a history of heart disease, lung cancer, prostate cancer, Alzheimer's disease, and a long history of alcoholism. However, unlike some of my family members, I have absolutely no fear of developing, nor do I have signs of any of these diseases. Why, not? It is because I understand these diseases, in the overwhelming majority of cases, are not genetically-determined diseases. They are lifestyle, or choice-based diseases.

While it may be true and even verifiable that I possess a specific "prostate cancer" or "Alzheimer's" gene, that in no way, means I am going to develop these diseases. It simply means if I *choose* to live in an unhealthy fashion, there is a *chance* I *could* develop these diseases. If I make poor health decisions throughout my life there is a *greater* chance I will develop these diseases than if I make healthy decisions.

Similarly, I am not likely to suddenly, one day become an alcoholic, even if I do possess an alcoholism gene. That is something I must *choose* to do. *Think* about it. Do you *really* think having an alcoholism gene means you will be an alcoholic? *Think*. Were you an alcoholic when you were seven years old? No? Why, not? It's because you probably didn't have easy access to alcohol. If alcoholism were genetic, doesn't it stand to reason there would be a bunch of alcoholic infants and children running around the world screaming at their parents for more alcohol in their bottles and juice boxes? If alcoholism is genetic, why is it the disease usually doesn't manifest until late teenage years or adulthood when most people are able to access alcohol? The *honest* answer is because alcoholism is a *choice*, a learned behavior in its initiation, not a genetic disease. Calling alcoholism a disease is as ridiculous as calling compulsive shopping a disease.

Furthermore, merely having a "history" of a disease in the family is not evidence any given disease is "genetic." I may have a "history" of an uncle and a brother who each won the lottery at one time in their lives, but that in no way suggests I have a "genetic" predisposition for winning the lottery. Just because my brother and uncle each won the lottery doesn't increase the likelihood I will win the lottery. But, if I *choose* to play the lottery, it does!

Beliefs Can Trigger Genetics

Belief can activate or deactivate a gene's expression. A good friend of mine literally watched his 56-year-old father drop dead of a heart attack. Ever since then, my friend has *believed* he, too, will probably die in his mid-fifties. He talks like he will, believes it, and what do you know? He behaves like it! My friend is a victim of what Stephen Covey jokingly calls genetic determinism.

Because my friend lives life at a fairly low level of health awareness and is a strong believer in genetic mysticism, he is convinced he won't live much longer than his father did. Interestingly, his mother lived into her eighties, so I'm not quite sure why he is so adamant about taking after his father. Perhaps because he connects with his father more by virtue of his gender.

My friend is sending die messages to his body. He may have a genetic predisposition for heart disease; however he could make wiser health choices than his father did. He could keep his weight in check, eat more organic foods, exercise more, better handle emotional stress, and he could *intend* to live much longer. But, he doesn't. The beliefs he *chooses* daily set him on a course similar to his father's. Can you see how his beliefs can activate and/or accelerate his genetic predispositions?

At this point some people might tell me, "Well, that's not fair. You can't control your beliefs." What makes you say that? I choose my beliefs all the time. And, so do you! *Think* about it. How do people acquire their religious beliefs? In most cases they choose them. Perhaps they don't think they choose them. Perhaps they grew up in a household of a particular faith. But once they grow up and learn to think for themselves, they can choose not to believe can't they?

You're Probably Not an Exception

It has been proposed by research that genetics, by itself, only accounts for about 5% of most diseases and conditions, including obesity. However, my experience has been that 95% of obese people are absolutely convinced their obesity is due to their genetics. Why do the overwhelming majority of fat people think they all fall into that extreme minority of genetically-based obesity? Somehow, I don't think I could possibly personally know 95% of that 5%.

You see? It's dishonesty. Genetics provides a convenient excuse for those who do not want to change. Rather than recognize it is their *choices* that make them sick and fat, it's simply easier to attribute their illness or poor health to genetic mysticism.

~ 15 ~

BEING FAT IS A CHOICE

As we continue to spend some time here at The Honesty Point and appreciate its powerful perspective, we now must recognize that being fat is a choice. No, "Yeah, buts" about this, please. The longer you choose not to recognize being fat is a decision *you* make, the longer you will be fat. As discussed earlier, you may or may not recognize being fat as your *fault*, but, it is your *responsibility* to fix it. It is your responsibility to yourself, your relationship, your children, the rest of your family, and even your friends.

Being fat doesn't just hurt you. Yes, it affects to some extent nearly everyone else you care about. It makes your parents sad for you. It embarrasses your children and humiliates your spouse. It inhibits your ability to succeed in the workplace or business (studies document fat people often earn less and are overlooked for promotion). It also makes your friends uncomfortable around you because you often can't participate in some activities like hiking, or even walking around a city, because you're too fat to keep up.

The Honesty Diet

America's Largest Eating Disorder

In the last couple of decades, much attention has been focused on eating disorders. Most people would say the two main categories of eating disorders are anorexia and bulimia. However, anorexia and bulimia are only the two *most-recognized* eating disorders. The two main *categories* of eating disorders describe those who eat *too little* and those who eat *too much* – under-eating disorder and overeating disorders, if you will. Even though those who eat *too much* is a leading cause of preventable death and disease in the United States, those who eat too *little* are given a disproportionate and inappropriate amount of attention.

Accurate statistics for annual *deaths* caused by eating disorders are difficult to ascertain. However, it is safe to say the *ratio* of deaths caused by overeating disorders like obesity, compared to under-eating disorders like bulimia and anorexia, is somewhere in the neighborhood of one hundred to one (100:1). That is, for every *one* person who dies from an under-eating disorder like anorexia, *one hundred* people die from an overeating disorder. The ratio is completely disproportional. There is simply no question as to which eating disorder is more of a problem in this country. Yet so much attention and focus is placed on bulimia and anorexia. Only in America, the fattest country in the world, could we make such a big deal over people who eat *too little*! Only the fattest country in the world could be so obsessed with the handful of celebrities and the relatively small percentage of non-celebrities who appear to have under-eating disorders.

Obesity Is the Real Eating Disorder

Because of the devastating impact obesity has had on our healthcare system and the unfair burden it places on non-obese people's medical insurance premiums, I can actually appreciate, to some degree, the efforts of those with under-eating disorders. At least many of those with under-eating disorders are striving for something healthier – to weigh less! Please do not misunderstand or take this comment out of context. I am not dismissing the significant problem of under-eating disorders. Nor am I suggesting bulimia and anorexia are healthy ways of living. They're not. These *habits* are serious disorders warranting significant attention. However, statistically speaking, those who under-eat are much less likely to be sick and diseased than those who overeat. For us to over emphasize under-eating disorders, *at the expense of* the most common eating disorder – obesity – is like ignoring the big, fat, white elephant in the room (pun very much intended).

Studies have been done on various types of vertebrates – animals with spines like humans – which have demonstrated when fed less food, their lifespan *increases* substantially. Some by as much as 50%! Additionally, people and animals who do not overeat have a fraction of the disease and health problems and live a much higher quality of life than people and animals who overeat. Overall, those who under-eat are extraordinarily healthier than those who overeat.

Changing Standards

When I was growing up there was usually only *one* fat kid in the classroom, and it was he or she who was teased by others. Today, in many elementary classrooms across America, reports indicate it is not uncommon for almost half the class to be fat! Today, it is often the skinny kids who are teased. My, how times have changed for the worse.

I find it disturbing that fat children today often tease skinny children for being so skinny. After all, it is the fat children who are already showing signs of heart disease and are not going to live to be nearly as old as their parents. Interestingly enough, the fat kid in my class grew up to be an extremely healthy and fit person, largely because of the "bullying" he experienced from being teased during most of his adolescence. It provided him with the motivation to change. Today, there is little social incentive to not be fat. When everyone else around you is fat, too, why would you *want* to change? Ironically, you "fit" in!

"Come On... Live a Little."

I find it rather odd that people often say to me, "Come on, you have to *live* a little." This motto is just an excuse people use to get you to share in their weaknesses. Often it takes the form of cigarettes, chocolate, fatty foods, fast-foods, beer, or alcohol. Yet, all of the things I just listed have something in common. They all *harm* your health to one degree or another. Things that harm your health move you closer to *death* not life. Yet, these are the same people who say to me, "*Live* a little." As if consuming things that harm my body helps me *live* more. They don't. If you want to "live a little" try eating a vegetable, try getting a full night's sleep, or try going for a hike in the woods. These are *live* activities. The irony of the whole thing is that the way I eat and many of the other decisions I make don't allow me to live a *little*... They allow me to live *a lot*!

People who feel compelled tell you to "live a little" really are not saying that with any good intention toward you. It is really a defensive mechanism on their part meant to try to make themselves feel better for their less-than-ideal health choices. What they really mean is, "Come on, be like me. Be fat. Be lazy." What "live a little" also means is, "Please, don't make *me* feel bad for eating this." They try to make you feel bad about not wanting to put harmful substances into your body because they *intuitively* know they shouldn't be doing that either. They know they presently lack the fortitude to simply *decide* to refrain from eating unhealthful foods. But, you don't ever have to feel guilty about other people's choice to live poorly.

Sometimes people say to me, "You are no *fun* (as far as eating is concerned)." I don't get that. What's *fun* about being fat? What's *fun* about feeling stuffed? I'm not saying I don't *ever* overeat, eat a sweet, or a drink beer. I enjoy these things every *once in a while*. But today, most people indulge in these kinds of things daily. That is why the nation is so fat. If you are being *honest* with yourself, you'll know whether or not it is a good idea to participate in consuming these kinds of things. Just look in the mirror. If you're fit and healthy, then maybe it's OK. If you are fat-sick, then it probably isn't. See? It's easy. Just be honest.

The Two Types of Hunger

I recognize two types of hunger – *value-based hunger* and *quantity-based hunger*. The first is a natural, healthy phenomenon. The second is a product of a society that regularly practices gluttony. Value-based hunger means your body needs *nourishment*. Quantity-based hunger means your stomach *feels* empty and wants to experience the sensation of "fullness" at any cost.

Fullness is produced by a phenomenon called distention. Distention is a fancy way of saying "stomach stretching." Your stomach is only about the size of your closed fist. But how often do people eat meals larger than one fist? When your stomach stretches it sends signals to the brain saying you've eaten "too much." However, if you repeatedly stretch your stomach too often, by eating too much, your stomach no longer returns to its normal size. As a consequence, your brain loses its sense of proportionality and it can no longer properly determine what a healthy portion of food is. The result of this overstretching is your body "thinks" it needs more food than it really does.

Rapid Weight Loss Is *Never* Healthy

Excessive stomach stretching has become so chronic and so common in our society it has led to the invention of a series of surgical procedures, sometimes generally referred to by the public as "stomach stapling." In short, these procedures, more or less, "staple" or otherwise restrict parts of your overstretched stomach, thus creating a smaller stomach so when you eat you feel "full" sooner. The intent is to *artificially* return the stomach to the size of a *normal* or even smaller-than-normal person's. The end result is *rapid* weight loss. Because you can't eat as much as you did before, you can't help but lose weight rapidly.

There is only one huge problem with this procedure. It radically *deforms* your body! You end up looking like a monster. These procedures can cause such dramatic and rapid weight loss that your over-stretched skin (ultimately caused from overstretching your stomach) cannot retract at the same rate as your weight loss. As a result, your body *permanently* ends up looking like a pile of wet laundry! Your body *literally* looks like a melted candle. You may weigh less, but you look *worse* than ever. I liken these procedures to anorexia. It works, but it sure as hell isn't healthy.

The other downside to this approach is you don't solve the problem. You are still not *nourishing* your body. Indeed, you may be eating a lot *less* stuff, but that doesn't mean you are *nourishing* your body any more than before. In fact, unless you radically change the foods you *choose* to eat, you are probably nourishing your body *less*. The *only* societal benefit of the invention of surgical stomach stapling procedures is *it has proven beyond a shadow of a doubt* that the primary reason why Americans are so fat is simply because they eat too much! It's not fast-food's fault. It is not soft drinks' fault. It is *our* fault.

Unless you are so morbidly obese you pose an immediate risk to yourself, you probably don't need this kind of procedure. Rapid weight loss is *never* healthy. So stop trying to do it! You didn't get fat overnight, did you? Then why are you looking to get thin overnight? Rapid weight loss of any kind is a disease in and of itself – even when a result of surgery. If rapid weight loss were healthy, then your skin wouldn't look like a melted candle. If rapid weight loss were healthy, your skin would retract proportionally. With a more honest awareness, losing weight is actually very simple. You can get the same benefits, and I would even argue you can get *better*, healthier benefits without surgery simply by teaching yourself not to stretch your stomach when you eat.

One of the best techniques for not overeating and feeling "full" is simply to slow down. Occupy yourself with some other task while eating if you have to, but slow down! Typically, it can take fifteen or twenty minutes for the nerve centers in the stomach to inform the brain through hormone secretion that the stomach is satisfied. If you shove your entire dinner in your stomach in just a few minutes you stretch your stomach, spike your insulin and blood sugar levels, and ultimately, you get fatter.

"Full" Means Failure

The way you know you've stretched your stomach, i.e. you've eaten "too much," is if you have that "full" feeling. Most people think the "full" sensation means that you've eaten "enough." We even say things like, "Well, I've had *enough*. I feel *full*, now." But, in reality, "full" means you've eaten "too much." A feeling of "fullness" means you are on your way to gaining weight.

> *Fullness means failure. If you feel "full" you are getting fatter.*

I know there is a social camaraderie associated with feelings of "fullness," especially around holiday meals like Thanksgiving, Easter, and Christmas. There exists a sense of success or completion, pride — a patting of the belly, a loosening of the pants. This would be OK if these were the only occasions we indulged like this. Unfortunately, it isn't. Most Americans do this several times per week. Some people do it at least once per day. Others still, do this at *every* meal!

Americans Are Starving!

Each year, many generous, thoughtful Americans send money to starving children in third-world countries. I commend them for this and think it is wonderful. However, I would offer for consideration that some of those "starving" children in third world countries are actually more "nourished" than many children in the United States. Just because we are fat, doesn't mean we are *nourished*.

In fact, the irony of the obesity epidemic in the United States is that the fattest nation on the planet isn't fat because they are over nourished. Quite to the contrary, America is the fattest nation on the planet because we are *starving*! That's right. Americans are so fat because they are chronically malnourished. Fat Americans are starving, starving for nutrition, that is. Nourishment is about *quality*, not quantity, of food.

I am convinced one of the primary reasons Americans eat too much food is because so much of the readily available food supply lacks any nutritional value. Let's say you eat a big fast-food meal containing no nutritional value and then feel hungry soon afterward. The reason is because you didn't *nourish* your body. So your body just continues to ask for nourishment by sending you more hunger sensations. It will do this until it gets what it needs. When people eat poorly all the time, the body never gets the nutrients it needs to thrive and function properly. So the body begins to panic. It begins to *store* energy as fat because the body is afraid it will *never* get any nourishment. It is a big, fat, vicious cycle (again, pun very much intended).

Indulgence Fat: An Energy Surplus

To make it easier to understand how and why fat accumulates in the body, I divide fat into two categories. The difference between these fats is not structural, but philosophical. That is, *why* they accumulate in the body. The first type I call *indulgence fat*. Indulgence fat is an energy surplus. That is, people with indulgence fat consume far more energy than they need or expend. Indulgence fat simply means eating *too much* and moving *too little*. This is the primary and most common mechanism resulting in obesity in the United States.

Toxicity Fat: The Junk Drawer

The second kind of fat is a more devastating kind called *toxicity fat*. Toxicity fat *compounds* and *amplifies* the effects of indulgence fat. Toxicity fat occurs when you eat foods chock full of unnatural substances, such as trans-fatty acids (a.k.a. "trans-fats"), steroid hormones, antibiotics, pesticides, herbicides, artificial preservatives, and toxic metals like mercury. Your body has tremendous difficulty breaking down these kinds of substances and burning them as energy. So, the body very intelligently *quarantines* these synthetic and/or toxic substances in a place where they will do the *least* amount of damage to your body – in your fat tissue. It is similar to the way health officials quickly quarantine an individual infected with a deadly, contagious disease to a place where the outbreak can be prevented from spreading and harming others.

For the most part, quarantining these substances neutralizes their toxicity, but you are still carrying them in your fat. I call this phenomenon "The Junk Drawer," because it is very much like the miscellaneous junk drawer you probably have somewhere in your home. It's the place where you collectively throw all the "junk" you can't find a place for anywhere else. The only problem is this junk drawer keeps getting bigger – much like many people's bellies and rear ends. When existing fat tissue fills up with these toxic substances, your body just makes more fat tissue to accommodate the next wave of toxins you consume.

> *"Why do we feed cows too sick to stand, to people who are too fat to walk?"*
>
> - Comedian, Bill Maher

The new awareness, then, is quite simple:

The more toxins you consume, the fatter you get.

Our bodies do have mechanisms for eliminating many of the toxic substances mentioned above. However, when we overwhelm these mechanisms by regularly consuming foods laden with these synthetic chemicals and pollutants, our bodies compensate by packing on the fat. If people only consumed these kinds of substances occasionally, we would probably fare OK. However, since most people choose to eat these substances daily, at almost every meal, our natural defense mechanisms are constantly being overwhelmed. While it is intelligent for the body to quarantine these substances in the fat tissue, the excessive consumption of these substances produces obesity and contributes to the thousands of annual deaths that result.

I am convinced the reason I did not gain a single pound of total body weight during my year of immobilization from my back injury (in fact, I lost weight) is because I didn't consume foods containing any of these toxic substances. It was not because of my *genetics*. I've been fat before, when I ate garbage. I did not gain any weight because of my *awareness* and my *choices*. After all, what is the likelihood I didn't gain weight because of some very fortunate genetics *and* I just also happened to be the kind of person who doesn't eat these toxins? Pretty slim, I think.

As you can see, even if you do not overeat, you could still gain toxicity fat because your body is *intelligently* trying to *neutralize* poisons you consume in your food. If you are having difficulty losing weight, and you are *honestly* not eating more than you should, you may want to consider exploring this idea of *toxicity fat* more carefully. It is possible your body is deliberating holding on to excess body fat as a way of defending itself against the long-term accumulation of chemical toxicity.

~ 16 ~

ADDICTION IS A CHOICE

What Is Addiction?

Contrary to what you may have been conditioned by society to believe, addiction is a perfectly *normal*, even favorable, human trait. Addiction means through the decisions you've consistently made, your body has developed the *perception* of a biochemical need for a substance or an activity and its associated *feelings*. You can be addicted to virtually anything, and this can work in your favor or against it. Addiction is a normal capacity *all* human beings possess and exhibit in one way or another. No one is immune from addiction.

Furthermore, addiction is *not* a disease. Addiction is always a *choice*. It is a biochemical phenomenon that, *no matter what*, initiates from choice. As we discussed in the chapter on genetics, it is our *choices* that largely determine what genes will or will not be expressed in a person's physiology. Even if you have an "addiction" gene, that doesn't make addiction a disease any more than my having a gene for blue eyes makes blue eyes a *disease*.

Addiction: A Powerful Tool

Humans are kings of addiction, but addictions aren't something we can or should have to fight. All we have to do to succeed in any venue is to choose our addictions carefully.

Addiction is a lot like financial debt. Financial debt can make you extremely rich or it can make you extremely poor. Most people *choose* to use financial debt to make themselves extremely poor. Others, like real estate investors, use financial debt to make themselves extraordinarily wealthy. Many real estate investors are *addicted* to making money, because doing so is so easy for them, and it provides them with massive wealth and an incredible lifestyle.

You see? Addiction is a powerful tool that can be used in healthy ways or unhealthy ways. Addiction isn't something to fear. Addiction is something to *use*, to *control*, and to cause you to become as healthy and fit as you want to be. Choose your addictions and let them work for you instead of against you.

Addiction Gets a Bad Rap

People tend to think addiction is *always* bad. That's wrong. Addiction can be a great tool and a great asset. The trick is to *consciously choose* your addictions wisely and not let them choose you.

For example, I would say I am *addicted* to organic food. I am addicted to organic food because of how organic food makes me *feel*. I deliberately *chose* this addiction. In the same way prescription drugs or junk food make other people *feel* good, organic foods make me feel good... *really* good! Organic foods make me feel so good that I don't quite feel myself when I have to eat something other than organic foods.

I know this may sound a bit strange to some, but it is no stranger than people who don't quite feel themselves if they don't get their morning cup of coffee and doughnut. I am so *addicted* to organic food that I am more than happy to pay a premium for organic foods; much like some drug addicts are willing to pay top dollar for their drug habit. I am also addicted to exercise and sunshine. I am so addicted to these things that I feel terrible if I don't get them almost daily. It is remarkably similar to the way fast-food junkies feel about their addictions. They *feel* terrible without them, but *feel* balanced, happy and safe when they do get them (at least for a little while). The difference is my addictions make me *healthier*. Most people's addictions make them sicker. I *consciously* choose my addictions, while others become addicts through unconscious choices.

Don't fight addiction. Use it to your advantage. Choose to become addicted to health.

What Are You Addicted To?

You know when you are addicted to something when you start to use language like, "I *need*..." instead of "I'd like." For example, "I *need* a cup of coffee." "I *need* a cigarette." "I *need* a cookie." These are all things that aren't *required* by the body, but many people think they can't function without them. Now, saying "I need oxygen" or "I need a glass of water" wouldn't be an addiction, because those are things required by the body.

However, when you believe you *need* things like coffee, cigarettes, beer, cookies, or fast-food to make your day work, then, you have evidence you are, in fact, addicted to those things. If your whole morning is thrown off by the fact that you didn't get a greasy egg sandwich, then you have a significant problem. If going cold turkey from a suspected addiction for just a few days or less causes you to have any trouble functioning or causes you any symptoms associated with withdrawal (like headache or anxiety), that, too, is an excellent indicator you are a junkie to that substance.

You can use this same technique to determine whether or not you are addicted to healthy things like exercise or nutrition, just as much as you can for bad things, like coffee. If you find yourself saying, "I *need* to go for a walk," or "I feel dehydrated, so I really *need* to eat some fruit" these, too, are addictions. However, they are addictions that make you healthier.

Here's another easy way to tell if you are addicted to something. If you notice, for instance, that just the *idea* of quitting something like coffee causes you *any* mental distress whatsoever, then you are probably addicted. If you firmly contend you are *not* addicted to a substance, then the idea of stopping for a few days or a week shouldn't scare you and shouldn't be difficult. If it is difficult, and if you are being *honest* with yourself, then you know you are addicted.

Addiction Is Not Genetic

Regardless of the presence or absence of an "alcohol" gene, a "fat" gene, a "violence" gene, or a "blame-others-for-everything-wrong-with-you" gene, the *expression* of many, if not most, genes begins with *choice*. That is why you must *choose* your addictions. Addiction isn't genetic. The biochemical reaction in your body for exercise is virtually the same as it is for heroin. The difference is some people *choose* to be in control of their addictions, and others *choose* to let their addictions control them.

As I mentioned earlier, there is a long history of alcoholism in my family. If several of my family members and I were subjected to formal genetic testing, I'm certain a so-called "alcoholism" gene would be found in all of us. Yet, none of my immediate family is an alcoholic. We are not alcoholics, *not* because we lack the gene for alcoholism, but because we *choose* not to be alcoholics – even though we all probably have the genetic capacity to be alcoholics.

In the overwhelming majority of cases, it is the *choice* to be or not to be an alcoholic that *expresses* an alcoholism gene. Despite having the gene for alcoholism, we make conscious daily choices keeping the gene from being expressed. Similarly, many people who do not possess the "alcoholism gene" are alcoholics. How's that possible if alcoholism is genetic?

People Are Addictive; Not Substances

In America, labeling substances and activities as "addictive" can almost be considered a popular pastime. Alcohol is addictive; prescription drugs are addictive; tobacco is addictive; video games are addictive; pornography is addictive, etc. I most adamantly disagree. *Things* are not addictive. *People* are addictive.

Anybody can become addicted to anything. There exists a widely popular perception that only "bad" things can be addictive. That is completely untrue. People can become addicted to healthy or "good" things just as easily. People can also become addicted to benign things like watching television or cleaning the house. Sometimes people can become addicted to healthy things that if abused can turn into unhealthy things. For example, there are some people, albeit very few, who are addicted to exercise to the point where they harm themselves. Now, being addicted to exercise is a good thing. But too much of anything can become a bad thing. Exercising to the point of harming oneself (called anorexia athletic) is obviously a bad thing. These individuals, frequently women, are so obsessed with losing weight that they exercise excessively. This is different than the much more common form of anorexia, anorexia nervosa, in which people simply refuse to eat.

There is a movement in society to punish companies

like fast-food restaurants and tobacco companies that produce unhealthy products. We have a tendency to blame our health problems on them. This, once again, reminds me of the Stephen Covey quote: "If you think the problem is outside of yourself, *that*, in and of itself, is the *real* problem." Fast-food restaurants and tobacco companies are things *outside of ourselves*. That is why we like to blame them for our health problems. Our *unwillingness* to be honest, to look inward and take control, to assume power and responsibility, is what truly makes us unhealthy. In the case of fast-food restaurants, which are probably the biggest vice among Americans today, the food, itself, is not addictive. The customers are! The customers are adversely *addictive* people. People are addictive, not foods and not drugs.

The Addiction Awareness

I have almost come to blows with some people about my next assertion. It is an awareness many people find difficult to accept, because it directly conflicts with one's physical senses. Here it is:

For those of you who say you "need" your addictions, I assert you do not really "like" them. You do not really "like" coffee, you do not really "like" beer, and you do not really "like" candy, soda, or chocolate. You only *think* you do! Now I know this may sound a bit absurd. In fact, I can already hear many of you protesting. "What do you mean I don't like coffee? I *love* my coffee!" Or, "I'm not addicted to coffee, I just enjoy it!" While this can be true, usually it isn't. I would suggest you don't honestly enjoy coffee. You only *think* you do because of your *addiction*.

While you may enjoy part of the experience of coffee, such as the warmth, the ritual, and the way its stimulating caffeine can make you *feel*, it is doubtful you actually *like* the way it tastes. Its taste is less a matter of what your body "likes" and is more a function of what your body has become used to. I mean, come on. Be honest. Coffee tastes like putrid dirty water. Just try giving some to a baby and listen to her cry. If you don't believe me, consider this: Do you drink coffee black? Or do you dress it up with sugar, milk, whipped cream, and syrup flavors? If you do dress it up, *why* do you dress it up? It's because coffee fundamentally tastes like garbage to most people! Especially when a person *first begins* to drink it!

Think about that. How old were you when you had your first cup of coffee? Did it honestly taste good? Or, did you just really "need" it? Putting sugar in coffee makes it barely tolerable. We only *think* sweetened coffee tastes good because of how it makes us *feel*, not because of how it *tastes*. We only *think* coffee tastes good after our brain has *altered our perception* of the taste. If you do drink coffee black, then it's likely you're even *more* addicted than most other people.

Is this a problem? I think so. Coffee temporarily hardens the coronary arteries of the heart. It also drains the adrenal glands and probably causes numerous other health problems. If we are not careful about consciously choosing our addictions for our betterment, we may harm ourselves.

Because of the "good" feelings associated with drinking coffee, the body's nervous system reassigns the *perception* of pleasure signals to that substance. For example, coffee, in and of itself, tastes terrible, but because we *associate* pleasurable or socially-necessary *feelings* with coffee, like alertness, productivity, and energy, our nervous systems *assume* it is something we *need*, or something we *want*. Our bodies then create the cyclical, biochemical reactions we call cravings to meet the new need – the addiction – even if the substance is harmful to our health.

This is true with coffee, alcohol, candy, and fast-food, just as much as it is with heroin, crack, and prescription medications. Of course, the healthy and natural way to get the *same* feelings coffee *artificially* provides is to *value* sleep, exercise, nutrition, and stress reduction. These choices – these habits – provide the same perceived benefits as coffee, but don't harm our health. In fact, they do quite the opposite. They make us healthier and happier. These healthy addictions follow the same biochemical mechanism as the coffee addiction or any other addiction. They are equally addictive. But they build up health as opposed to breaking it down.

> *"The chains of habit are too weak to be felt, until they are too strong to be broken."*
>
> – English Author, Samuel Johnson

Don't Take Advice From Fat Doctors!

This exact phenomenon will also occur if you give a baby a sip of wine. A baby will start to cry, because wine tastes terrible. People only like wine because of the *effect* the alcohol has on their body. How do I know this is true? Alcoholic wine and beer vastly outsells nonalcoholic, wine and beer. If wine and beer were pleasant-tasting drinks, then there would be no need for their alcohol content. The same would apply to caffeinated sodas. While to some people soda may taste sweet and therefore good, why do caffeinated sodas far outsell decaffeinated sodas? It is because of the *addiction* people have to caffeine.

For example, I think most people would agree that repeatedly pressing a red-hot cattle iron against your thigh would be pretty painful. However, let's say in a crazy laboratory experiment, electrodes were hooked up to the brain that created orgasmic sensations throughout your entire body that lasted for 15 minutes *every time* your thigh was branded with that red-hot cattle iron. Through repetition, you could eventually be conditioned to associate the orgasmic feelings to the cattle iron.

This is just plain old Pavlovian classical conditioning. After being conditioned, you would adamantly swear you really do like the cattle iron being pressed against your thigh because of the euphoric way it makes you *feel*. Your nervous system has linked the hot cattle iron and the orgasmic feelings to each other in an "apparent" cause-and-effect relationship. Your nervous system now "thinks" it likes the hot cattle iron pressed against your thigh.

This is the *exact* mechanism by which coffee, soda,

alcohol, cigarettes, fast-food, or junk food work. You don't really "like" these things; you just "think" you do because of the chemically-induced, addictive *feelings* you have attributed to these substances.

The proof of this addiction can be illustrated by the attitude of defensiveness in those who are accused of being coffee addicts, chocolate addicts, or whatever. Merely suggesting to these people they stop using a substance for even a short period of time sends them into a verbal tirade. Their eyes widen, their voice rises in pitch and volume, and they begin speaking faster. They tend to become agitated, vehemently defend their habit, and deny their addiction. The more vehemently they react to the suggestion, the more addicted to the substance they are. The suggestion to stop using the substance instills fear in them. If they weren't addicted, there would be no fear of the suggestion. If they weren't addicted, they could, at the very least, entertain and contemplate the notion. But, more often than not, these addicts can't even do that.

How does this suggestion sound to you? Are you experiencing any feelings of fear, or are you rejecting this suggestion outright? If so, you are probably addicted to coffee or something else yourself.

In the beginning of this book, I mentioned there would be times where something The Honesty Diet suggests will have to be *experienced* in order to be understood. This chapter may be one of those times for you. If you have *chosen* an addiction to junk food, coffee or something else that harms your health, it's unlikely I'll be able to "sell you" or convince you of this awareness purely by written word. You can only really understand what I'm saying through experience. If you'll try this, I think you will find as you choose to make healthier decisions, you'll *lose* your taste for junk foods. I did. So can you.

Addiction is learned. Fortunately, addiction can also be unlearned. Whatever the addiction, healthy or unhealthy, if you stop *doing* it, you gradually *lose* the craving *for* it. Most people have this backwards. They think if they could just stop the craving, they could break the habit. But, the truth is it works the other way around. In order to understand and embrace this awareness you have to *acknowledge* you are addicted to it. You have to *want* to no longer be an addict. And, you have to *decide* to make different decisions to break this adverse addiction. Our new awareness, then, is:

***You don't really like your vices,
you only think you do.***

~ 17 ~

LONGEVITY IS A CHOICE

Longevity = Expectation x Choices x Change

Longevity Is a Choice

Accidents aside, how old you live to be is very much *your* choice. Genetics, as we have already discussed in an earlier chapter, actually play very little role in your health. I contend they also play very little role in how *long* you live. In my opinion, the biggest factor in how long you live is *choice*. People who *decide* (either consciously or unconsciously) to live to be 100 years old make daily choices that work toward that specific age goal. Similarly, people who decide to live to be only 60 years old also make daily choices that work toward *that* specific age goal. These two sets of choices are often just very different from one another. Again, these choices are not necessarily *conscious* choices. They may be choices that were socially conditioned into us by others and by our experiences in our environment.

For example, a man may say to himself and to others he wants to live to be 100 years old, but then his *choices* and *decisions* suggest otherwise. He may *choose* to smoke, not to exercise often, not to sleep well, and subsequently he may die at age 60. Even though he may have *said* he wanted to live to be 100 years old, he clearly did not *believe* it. If he did believe it, if he did value living to be 100, he would have made different choices to increase the likelihood of achieving that age. Actions do speak louder than words.

As humans, we have a bad tendency to associate causality to events, occurrences, and activities, that in fact bear no relation to each other at all. That is, people often choose to believe things that aren't really true regardless of the presence or absence of evidence. For example, in the 1400s Europeans were conditioned to believe the world was flat. There was no *evidence* of such, but people still *believed* it. Today, people have been socially conditioned to believe pharmaceutical drugs make us healthy. Although if that were true, Americans, who consume more pharmaceutical drugs than any other people, would be the healthiest people on the planet. They're not. Despite an overwhelming lack of evidence, the belief that pharmaceuticals make us healthy persists.

Today, people also collectively believe age 75, for example, is "old" and near the end of a human's lifespan. This, like anything else, can be a conscious or subconscious belief, but is more often than not subconscious social conditioning.

Consider people who consciously or subconsciously believe they will only live to be in their sixties or seventies. What kinds of things do they say to themselves? They may say, "What does it matter if I exercise or not? I'm already old." What kinds of food choices do they make? "Hey, I can eat this junk. That's why I take cholesterol medication, isn't it? So I can eat garbage like this!"

At the time of this writing, average US life expectancy is in the mid-to-late seventies. Many people think 75 years is old. Others, such as me, are less impressed with this statistic. Many physiologists contend the human body is designed to live 120 to 150 years or more. Others scoff at this contention. But is it really unreasonable to think 120 to 150 years-old is unachievable?

Jeanne Louise Calment died in 1997 at the confirmed age of 122 years old. This is only 23% shy of the 150 years old "limit" some physiologists assert. Imagine making the foolish statement 200 years ago (when average life expectancy was 40) that people would never live to be 51 years old (only 23% longer). What if 200 years ago you had told people average life expectancy would be near 80 by the 21st century? An almost 100% increase! Don't you think they would have laughed at you? Well, you would have been right. They would have been wrong… and dead. So let's not repeat the past and completely dismiss out of hand this notion of living 120 to 150 years.

If we are only living to our mid-seventies, then we are currently only about 50% successful in terms of longevity. Honestly, that really sucks. But who knows? Perhaps, by the time you're reading this book average US life expectancy is 100 years old or more.

Expectancy

Despite the poor success rate, the average life expectancy in the United States has increased steadily for the past 200 years or so. Why? It certainly isn't because of medical advances. Several researchers and studies have shown the increase in average life expectancy is primarily due to improved sanitation and hygiene, and not medical advances.

I contend the *most* important factor affecting average life expectancy is *expectancy*. What I mean by this is I think there is a socially-conditioned expectation for most to live longer than previous generations. However, while they psychologically expect to live longer, they do not expect to live *that* much longer. Hence, if someone's parents lived to be 75 then we have a tendency to *expect* to live to be a little bit longer, like maybe 79. But very few of us would *expect* to live to be 120 years old or more. Why? I'm not sure. Maybe it is some bizarre form of psychological deference or guilt that we shouldn't live to be *that* much older than our parents. Maybe, in some way, we subconsciously think it would be disrespectful or unfair to live a lot longer than our parents did. I *expect* to live at least 120 years because that is what the physiologists say the human body is designed for. As a result of this *belief*, I *try* to make daily health choices I think are congruent with this expectation.

So where am I going with this? Why introduce this concept of socially-conditioned or society-influenced longevity? It's because I firmly contend the reason why most of us only live to about 50% of our lifespan potential is because that is what we *see* and *experience* all around us every day. What we see and experience everyday significantly affects and influences our beliefs, expectations, and the daily choices we make about our own health and longevity. If these choices are not made with the highest level of health awareness, we, in essence, fulfill our socially-conditioned lifespan expectations, which for most of us is currently around the end of our eighth decade. That is, if we see most of our peers only living to their mid-seventies, then we *subconsciously* expect and, therefore, choose to *only* live to our mid-seventies, as well. This subconscious assumption, and therefore expectation to only live to be in our mid-seventies, alters the choices we make on a daily basis.

Currently, there are almost 500,000 people living on the planet over 100 years old, referred to as centenarians. Japan alone has more than 60,000 of them. So, do you still think 75 is a "ripe" old age?

Be Careful... Your Body Is Listening

This subconscious expectation also affects the language we use with others and even the things we say to ourselves. I hear people in their early fifties say things about how "old" they are getting. "I can't do that anymore. I'm getting old!" Here's a little secret: while the body is incredibly intelligent, it doesn't know how to count. It doesn't *really* know how old it actually is. But, if you say, think and act as though 50 is "old," that is *exactly* how your body will respond – like an old person! If you are going to moan and groan at age 50, what do you think life is going to be like for the next 25 years or so? Pretty miserable I would contend. I've never heard someone say at 85 years old they thought they would only live to be 65. On the other hand, I can't recall someone who bitches and moans at 65 ever reach 85!

Your Body Understands Adjectives

While your body can't really count, it does understand adjectives. Remember: your body is a computer and only does what it is told. When you say, "I'm tired." That usually isn't a description of how you feel *physically*. It is usually a description of how you feel *mentally*. Instead, the body interprets such a statement as a *command*, and hence, responds accordingly.

One of my grandmothers used to make what I considered rather strange statements whenever she was asked a question she didn't understand. Instead of saying, "I don't understand what you mean. Could you explain that to me?" she would preface every answer with "I'm old!" It would sound something like this: "I'm old. I can't do that anymore." Or, "I'm old. That isn't important to me anymore." Or, "I'm old. I can't learn how to use a computer." What kind of message does "I'm old" give to the body? One of *life* or one of *death*? Do statements like these tell your body – your only asset – to grow or to die? Not surprisingly, in her mid-eighties, my grandmother "suddenly" developed Alzheimer's disease. Coincidence? I don't think so. To me there seems to be quite the self-fulfilling prophecy occurring here.

We must never forget our bodies function exactly like computers! They do not think for themselves, *they only do what they are told*. If you tell your body to *die*, that is exactly what it does. Similarly, if you tell your body to *live*, more often than not, that is exactly what it does, too.

I firmly contend people make health decisions according to how long they *believe* they are going to live. Some people may even profess their philosophy or make other proclamations aloud and in front of people by saying things like, "Life is short!" while drinking their 4th cup of oversized coffee or single-handedly finishing off an entire pizza. Others say things like, "I'll get all the sleep I need when I'm dead" not quite realizing such a statement is, in fact, expediting their eternal dirt nap.

Unless you come to recognize the awareness that our *expectations* for longevity originate from our subconscious and socially-conditioned observations, you, too, will likely be a victim of social conditioning. That is why I strongly recommend you choose to live to be as old as you *want* to be. If that is 150 years old or more... great! If you only *want* to live to be 75, that is OK, too. However, understand that if you choose to live significantly above the current average life expectancy, you must *believe* it in your mind. Only through *belief* will you *choose* to act upon your *belief* – your longevity goal – and do you stand a much greater chance of achieving that goal.

Action Is Evidence of Belief

So how do you know if you really *believe* and expect to live to be 100 or one 150? How do you know you aren't just pretending? That's an easy question to answer. If you *act* upon your belief! Action is *evidence* of belief. Just as action is evidence of *decision,* action is also evidence of belief. You will not *act* upon things you *don't* believe in. If you recall, that is also how we determined our values in an earlier chapter. The things we *do* are the things we *value*. Similarly, the things we *do* are the things we *believe*. If you *value* a belief or an expectation, then you will *act* upon it. If you don't act upon it, then you don't really believe or expect something. For example, if you expect to live to be 100 *and* you believe you want to live to be 100 then you probably recognize how important it is to exercise your mind and body daily – to take care of your only asset, your only vehicle. However, if you don't really believe you will live to be 100, you won't exercise every day. You'll come up with other things you think are more urgent, thereby fulfilling your *real* belief that you will probably only live to be in your mid-seventies like everyone else.

But What If I Don't Believe?

It can work the other way, too. You can *learn to believe* or *learn to expect* something you want simply by acting upon it *until* you believe it. Remember from earlier in the book that some things must be experienced for them to be learned. This is another one of those situations for many people. For example, let's say you are overweight and don't believe you can become fit. That belief can change in a very short period of time *if* you act *in spite of your disbelief*. By going to the gym three to four times per week for just a few weeks and getting even the smallest result like losing two pounds or even just increasing your energy level a bit, you will quickly adopt the belief you seek that you *can* become fit.

Here is the key. You can't just say it. You have to mean it, and taking *action* upon a belief or a desired belief is the *proof* of the belief. That is how *choice* effects longevity. If you really want to live to be 150 or more, you must expect it. You must decide it. You must believe it. You must *act* upon it. Then and only then will you actually have a shot at attaining it!

> *"Whether a man believes he can or believes he can't... he's right!"*
>
> – Benjamin Franklin

All that will have to occur before people start living to 150 years old is to see it happen once. In 1954, Roger Bannister, a British medical student became the first person documented to break the four-minute mile. Up until then it was *believed* (some erroneously called it a scientific "fact") a human being couldn't run a mile in less than four minutes. But guess what happened within a short time of word getting out that Roger Bannister had,

Don't Take Advice From Fat Doctors!

indeed, run a mile in less than four minutes? That's right. A bunch of other people "suddenly" broke the four-minute mile barrier, as well. How is this possible? Quite simply, there was no *evidence* a human couldn't run a four-minute mile, there was only a collective *belief* it couldn't be done. This is a perfect example of social conditioning – the mere belief something couldn't be done actually prevented it from being done. That is, until Roger Bannister *chose* to do it!

There is a fun, old story suggesting, from a physics point of view, that bees shouldn't be able to fly. Mechanically it was impossible. Of course, this was a silly assertion by physicists since bees do fly. The punch line of the story is: "Apparently, someone forgot to tell the bees they can't fly." I think a more accurate assertion would have been, "We humans are not smart enough yet to understand how bees fly." When it comes to longevity, you may want to keep stories like these in mind.

Objections to Longevity

Many people object, "Who wants to be that old and *decrepit*? This, too, is just a socially-conditioned belief. The only reason why you believe 150 years old has to mean decrepit is because you've never seen a vibrant, healthy 150-year-old. Does that mean it is not possible? One hundred years ago nobody had ever seen a cell phone. Does that mean it wasn't possible? Less than 40 years ago it wasn't possible to walk on the moon, yet it's now been done. Because of the way most people in their seventies look and feel today, people are afraid to imagine the way they might look like and feel like at 150. I think this fear is unfounded. People in their seventies today look the way they *should* look and feel at 150 years! Today, we just age faster than we should because we make choices congruent with the socially-conditioned *expectation* of living to our seventies.

Another common objection is "Who wants to be that old and alone? All of my friends would be dead." That would only be true if you stopped making friends. And, why would you do that? This is, again, a function of social conditioning. Just because you've never experienced something doesn't mean it isn't true. The absence of proof is not the absence of truth. If you *think* about it, isn't it kind of arrogant to assume that just because *you* haven't experienced something, it couldn't be true? People who lived 200 years ago never ever expected to live to their seventies because they rarely saw someone who did. If you *think* about it, it isn't really that far a stretch to imagine ourselves living to be 110 or more. In fact, dozens of people all over the world have lived to be that old already. Raise your awareness about longevity and transcend this social programming. It may be causing you to miss out on at least half of your life!

On many occasions I have witnessed people I care very much about justify their bad choices with their age. "I don't need to fit into a bathing suit anymore, I'm over 50!" Or, "I'm going to eat this unhealthy food because I'm already 60. What harm is it going to do to me?" These kinds of statements all have a subtle underlying presupposition that people are going to be dying soon. Subconsciously, they are saying to themselves something like, "*Well, my Dad died when he was 71. I'm 61 now, so I probably don't have more than 10 years left, so why not booze it up, drink too much coffee, and eat junk food?*" Now, were it not for these erroneous thoughts of one's destiny, a person may live to be 100 or even 120, but they most certainly will not if they subconsciously feed their body – if they feed their computer – with instructions like, "Please die around age 71!"

Regardless of what age we are now, we all are affected by these subconscious, socially-conditioned beliefs to one extent or another. Sometimes it takes the form of beliefs like, "I don't have to look attractive anymore. After all, I'm married." It is these same people who then are surprised and depressed when they can't find anyone to even look at them after their spouse left them for someone with a greater sense of self-worth and self-respect. Others might say, "I don't have to be fit anymore. After all, I'm a mom. I had children, which wrecked my body." They might be surprised then when their husband doesn't want to touch them in an intimate way. Of course, they also ignore the fact that millions of women have children and get right back into shape almost immediately. It isn't because of their genetics. It is because they *chose* not to let having kids be an excuse for slothfulness.

Longevity Requires Purpose

A love for life is a prerequisite for longevity. I rarely meet someone in their eighties or nineties who isn't *excited* about life. If you love life and want more of it, then you probably already know you are going to need a healthy, vibrant, functioning body in order to experience it. Many people don't want to live very long – and although I think that's sad, there is nothing wrong with that. People who don't love life often don't care how long they live. They just sort of live life with a plan of grow up, work for 40 years, retire for 10 years, then die. Again, there is nothing wrong with this attitude. However, I think if more people would recognize longevity is a function of *choice* (i.e. behavior), and not a function of *chance* (i.e. genetics), they may reconsider examining this low level of awareness they have about their longevity. For most people, living to be in their seventies is just a function of automated, social conditioning.

Do you *want* to live to be 120? *Why* do you want to live to be 120? Do you want to dance with your great-granddaughter at her wedding? Would that be meaningful to you? What about living for many decades in dozens of different countries? How about learning dozens of foreign languages? Is there a worthwhile political cause you'd like to see fulfilled? What else? What else would be meaningful to you?

Comedian and entertainer, George Burns booked performances until he was 100 years old. And that is also *exactly* how long he lived to be. He died shortly after turning 100. George's purpose was to entertain the world. If you're going to intend and expect to live to be well over 100 years old you're going to need a reason, a purpose. Everybody has a life purpose, but for too many it is often a socially-conditioned purpose – one with a very low level of awareness. Most people live life with a purpose of reaching retirement, playing some golf, and then dying around 70 or 75. That's not really much of a purpose, is it? That is why, I think, most people currently live to only 50% of their physical lifespan capacity. They have no real awareness about their potential. They have no purpose.

A Willingness to Change and Grow

Of course, you can't *stop* aging (Or, perhaps that is just *my* brain washing and socially-conditioned belief?), but you certainly can slow it down substantially. In addition to *expectation*, what also causes people to become old is their *unwillingness* to keep growing. As soon as you stop growing, you get old. Health and fitness expert, Jack LaLane (age 92 at the time of this writing) says the secret to staying healthy and alive is to keep moving. Life is motion, and motion means change. So, deciding to not stop growing is one way to dramatically slow down aging. I'm not just speaking metaphorically, either. I mean this quite literally. Pretend for a moment you are a vat of freshly-poured concrete. When the concrete hardens, you're dead. The longer you stir it, the longer you disturb it, the longer you move the poured concrete, the longer it takes to harden and the longer you live.

Stay Away from the "Good ol' Days"

Don't let your mind get stuck in a "good ol' days" way of thinking. If you do, your body will age rapidly. The "good ol' days" way of thinking is different for everyone. For some it was a high school championship football

The Honesty Diet

game or winning title of Prom Queen 30 years ago. For others, it was playing in a rock band in New York City in their twenties. What is the best, most memorable period in your life? If it isn't today, if it isn't right now, then you're probably getting older much sooner than you should. Today or even tomorrow should always be the best day of your life. If all you have to talk about are stories from high school or your trip to Europe from 15 years ago, then you are growing old... fast.

I have found two of the first physical signs a person is getting old is not aches and pains or wrinkles, but 1) a reluctance to change their *hairstyle* and 2) a tendency to only connect with *music* from their past. I know these things sound a bit silly. However, I really think they are significant. Symbols like these, and there are many more, represent an *attachment* to the past. They are symbols of what we perceive to be a better time in our lives.

A few years ago, I caught myself only listening to a kind of music I associate with an exciting period in my life. I even caught myself saying things "old" people say like, "Today's music isn't any good. It's nothing like it was twenty years ago." When I realized what I had said – when I realized I was sounding "old" – I decided to go find some new contemporary music I liked. To my surprise, I discovered dozens of great, contemporary artists that are just fantastic. Much of it is even better than the older music I had so much connected with. Now, I have a whole new genre of music that really gets me going.

It's not about trying to be younger than you are. It's about continuously choosing to live in the *present* and not defining your self-image with something of the past. The more you connect with the past, the more you *become* the past. When you think of yourself as a relic, you become one physically.

What's the Worst That Could Happen?

What is the worst thing that could happen by choosing to live to 120 - 150 years old? You might not? So what? Maybe by setting the *expectation* to live to be 120 years old you die at 103 instead. So you didn't achieve your goal. What do you care? You're dead anyway! But, if you hadn't set the *expectation* and instead chose to just follow your social conditioning – only believing you'd live to be of average age – you probably would have died around 75. Twenty-eight years! That's a big difference!

> *"Plan for life as though you are never going to die, and live life as though you might die tomorrow."*
>
> – unknown

Longevity and Finances

I think some people *choose* to die much earlier than they physically would have had to because they don't think they have the finances to sustain them to age 100 or more. This too, is an erroneous belief derived from social conditioning that affected people's financial discipline and financial decisions throughout their entire lives. If they had behaved as though they *intended* to live to be 150 years old, you bet their financial *choices* would have been very different and their results much better. For example, most people's retirement philosophy is to save up a nest egg and then live off of that nest egg for the rest of their lives. The problem with this way of thinking is it makes assumptions about when one is going to die. Perhaps subconsciously, many people die in accordance with their retirement plans so as not to upset or offend their financial advisors!

One time, someone told me about a conversation she had with a few of her friends. She shared with them a news story about an anti-aging researcher from Oxford University who had identified seven primary mechanisms of aging. As a result of his findings, he is certain humans will be capable of living to be 1,000 years old within the first half of the 21st century! "Isn't that great. Think of how much we could do!" However, one of the other women said, "Wow. That's depressing! Just think of how long you'd have to work!" That's right. This person would rather die more than 900 years early than work! To me, this sounds like a person with a very low level of *longevity* awareness. She also appears to have a very low level of *financial* awareness. Hopefully, if people were capable of living to be 1,000 years old they would learn enough about finances by, say, age 100 to live off of the their investments and not have to work for the rest of their life if they didn't want to.

~ 18 ~

CANCER IS A CHOICE

Welcome to what, for some, is absolutely the most offensive chapter of the book. Cancer is a choice. *Oh my god. He did not just say that, did he?* Yes, I did. However, if you've made it this far in the book you certainly know by now there is always a context to my intentionally provocative statements. This is no exception. I know some will be offended and upset with me for making such a statement, but this is true. Like most, I, too, have lost people I love to cancer. Perhaps I've even had my own experience with this issue. So please do not assume I am speaking out of naiveté.

In *most* cases, people *choose* to *grow* cancer. Certainly, they didn't choose to grow cancer deliberately. Remember: most of the choices people make on a daily basis are subconscious. But, ultimately, they choose to develop cancer slowly through their daily decisions. The choice not to exercise daily, the choice not to sleep enough, the choice not to insist upon being fit, the choice to not learn how to eat healthy, and the choice to suppress and not deal with adverse stresses in their lives. All of these daily decisions and many more, decade after decade culminate into a choice to grow cancer. Furthermore, let me be clear: children do not *choose* to grow cancer. That simply isn't what were discussing here, so don't try to "Yeah, but" your way out of this reality. We are specifically talking about autonomous adults who deliberately destroy their health through bad decisions.

I am by no means the first doctor to assert this. Best-selling author, Dr. Bernie Siegel has made similar assertions on the subject of people *choosing* cancer. I may present the concept differently than he has, but the fundamental principle is the same. Louise Hay and many others health authors have also written substantially on the subject of manifesting cancer through choice. Former Surgeons General, C. Everett Coop and Richard Carmona, in conjunction with much contemporary medical research, acknowledge most of the diseases affecting Americans, including cancer, are completely preventable if people would simply make better choices. So it's certainly not a new concept, but I recognize it can be an emotionally-challenging one.

Of course, these assertions are controversial and highly sensitive to many people. The idea that a person *chose* their cancer can be highly offensive, especially to those currently challenged with cancer or to those who have lost a loved one to cancer. However, as I suggest in an earlier chapter, nothing can change until we *perceive* a problem *differently* than we have in the past. Let's explore a somewhat literal, somewhat abstract exercise about how we perceive the disease of prostate cancer to see if we can philosophically illustrate some of the faulty thinking about cancer.

A middle-aged man is informed by his doctor he has a prostate cancer condition. Conventional treatment or medical "logic" could include removal of the prostate – a radical prostatectomy. It is logical to assume if you have prostate cancer and you subsequently remove the prostate, you would no longer have the cancer, right? Logically, it makes sense. However, in reality, it doesn't often work out that way. Research shows that *more than half* of all men with prostate cancer who elect to have their prostate removed, experience a recurrence within ten years. How is that possible if they had the prostate removed? Did you ever think about that? How could a person with prostate cancer have a recurrence of their cancer if they've already had their prostate removed? An oncologist's typical response is, "We must not have 'gotten it all' during surgery." I adamantly disagree with this highly-speculative conclusion. Remember from a previous chapter that disease is not a "thing." Similarly, cancer is not a "thing." Therefore, you can't remove "it" surgically. Disease and cancer are conditions – they are circumstances. They are not "things." I firmly contend the *real* reason most men who undergo a radical prostatectomy experience a recurrence of cancer is because the prostate was *not* the real problem. The *cancer condition* was the real problem, not the prostate. Please refer to the illustration below and really try to *think* about it.

The Honesty Diet

Let's say you have a:

PROSTATE CANCER CONDITION

Then, you decide to remove the prostate. What are you left with?

~~PROSTATE~~ CANCER CONDITION

That's right. You are still left with a *cancer condition*. That is, you still have the conditions *needed to grow cancer* to the surrounding organs and tissues. As some statistics show, removing the prostate doesn't necessarily solve the cancerous condition in the long run. This helps to illustrate it is not the diseased *organ* that is the problem. The problem was the *conditions* existing in the body which facilitated the development of cancer cells in the first place. And, those conditions that support the development of the cancer are called *choices*. Conditions are brought about through *choices*. Remember: the way we see the problem is the problem. Prostate cancer and many other diseases are diseases of *choice* and quite often, they are diseases of indulgence.

We know improper diet, stress, inadequate sleep and inadequate exercise all contribute to prostate cancer and most other cancers. That is not to say other things do not *also* cause prostate cancer. They do. However, without a doubt, most cancers, including prostate cancer, are caused by *choice*. Actually, prostate cancer appears to be one of the few studied cancers that may, in fact, have a genetic component to it. However, its genetic influence still appears to represent only a *minority* of total prostate cancer cases. *Choice* is the major factor.

Blaming Things Outside of Ourselves

Many prefer to blame their cancers on things outside of themselves like tobacco companies, industrial pollution, or even fast food restaurants. This is not a very honest approach to addressing one's health. People will frequently attribute blame to things they don't even know the first thing about. For example, as I am writing this chapter, I have come across an Internet news story about researchers who recently discovered that a small percentage of men with prostate cancer have high levels of a certain kind of virus in their prostate gland. Their assumption is the virus may cause the prostate cancer. Once again, we are trying to look for something *outside* of ourselves – something other than our own choices – as the cause for our problems. The story was trying to suggest, "It's not your fault. It's a virus!"

Has it ever been suggested that this particular virus proliferates within the prostate tissue of this small percentage of men *because* the prostate tissue has become susceptible and unhealthy through years of poor daily health choices? In my opinion, suggesting the presence of virus in the prostate is causative of the prostate cancer is just as silly as saying that flies found near garbage *caused* the garbage to be there in the first place.

Bacteria, viruses, fungi, parasites and alike, all have something in common. They all proliferate in an acid-rich environment – in a sick or *polluted* environment. If you make poor health choices, on a daily basis, for weeks, months, years, and decades, you create an acid-rich or "sick" environment in your physiology for things like viruses and bacteria to proliferate.

The idea of blaming prostate cancer on a virus is both attractive and convenient to many because it's something you are exposed to, not something you are not necessarily responsible for. This would imply your prostate cancer isn't really your fault. While it may be attractive and convenient to blame your cancer on something outside of yourself, that doesn't help you much, does it? On the other hand, once you acknowledge that it was your choices that created your predicament, you have the opportunity to reassume *power* and *control* to do something about it. Acknowledging responsibility empowers you and grants you the capacity to fix the problem. Denying responsibility for your disease dis-empowers you and leaves you merely a victim and a statistic.

A Short Story About Cancer

There once was a fat, 29-year-old woman named Gail who had the same body type as her mother and aunt, except Gail was much taller than both of them. Her aunt was diagnosed with having breast cancer at age thirty-five. At thirty-nine, Gail's mother was also diagnosed with breast cancer. Even Gail's grandmother had died of breast cancer in her early fifties. Gail was convinced she, too, would likely end up with breast cancer because of the strong family history of breast cancer.

Don't Take Advice From Fat Doctors!

One day, without informing her family, Gail went to go see a breast cancer specialist. "I'm really concerned I'm going to get breast cancer, too" she said. "I'm not sure what to do."

The doctor nodded understandingly and asked, "So, both your aunt *and* your mother were diagnosed with breast cancer in their thirties?"

"Yes," Gail answered.

"And, your grandmother? She died from breast cancer, as well?"

"Yes."

The doctor then explained to Gail her concerns were warranted. "Breast cancer does *run in families*," he said, "and, if you are really scared about *getting* breast cancer, you might want to seriously consider having both of your breasts removed now – just to be on the safe side."

"Yeah," Gail said. "I think that might be best… just to be safe." Gail went home depressed and even more scared than before. Having both of her breasts removed sounded really extreme to her. It definitely wasn't something she wanted to do but, "It's probably for the best," she said to herself.

Gail had scheduled the surgery for one month later. She couldn't do it right away because the doctor said Gail had to be completely off of cigarettes for at least three weeks before she could undergo the surgery. Gail complied, but still hadn't told her mother or her aunt why she had suddenly quit smoking. They were very proud of her for quitting, though. "Your mother and I have tried many times to quit smoking. We never could quit," her aunt told her.

The Honesty Diet

Two days before Gail's scheduled surgery, Gail was feeling very nervous. She finally decided to tell her mother and aunt about the preventive surgery she was about to undergo. Gail called her mother and aunt over to her house for some coffee and cake to break the news to them. "What!" exclaimed Gail's mother. "You're going to have your breasts removed! Why?"

"Because I'm scared! Because I don't want to end up with breast cancer like you two and Grandma. That's why!"

"Oh, Gail. How could you keep something like this from us? You should have told us right away what you were thinking of doing." Gail's aunt said.

"Why? I didn't see why I should unnecessarily worry you two," Gail said defensively.

The aunt looked at Gail's mother and said, "You have to tell her."

"Tell me what?" Gail said astonished.

Gail's mother closed her eyes as if in pain and after a few seconds said quietly to her daughter, "Gail, you're adopted."

"What?" Gail gasped.

"You're adopted," her mother repeated. "You're not going to get breast cancer. We don't share the same genes."

This young woman was going to remove her breasts to prevent a disease she believed was genetic – a disease she was absolutely convinced she was going to inherit. She agonized over it, living in absolute fear for years only to discover by chance that she bore no genetic relationship to her family members, three of whom had had breast cancer. Her oncologist never even bothered to ask her if

Don't Take Advice From Fat Doctors!

she was adopted. He just assumed since Gail had said *her* grandmother, mother, and aunt all had breast cancer, that she would probably get breast cancer, too. This is a pretty scary situation, isn't it?

But the story continues...

One year later Gail found a lump in her right breast. Shortly thereafter, she was diagnosed with an early stage breast cancer. "How could I have breast cancer? I'm adopted!" she asked the same oncologist.

"The gene probably runs in your birth mother's family, too" the doctor meekly offered. "That's the only explanation I can think of."

"I'm guess I'm just *unlucky*," Gail conceded. She then went ahead with a radical mastectomy of her right breast. She also had the left breast removed... just in case.

But the story continues, still...

After Gail had recovered from her preventive cancer treatment she became interested in finding out who her birth mother was and how her birth mother had handled breast cancer herself. Gail hired a private investigator to track down her birth mother. He couldn't find Gail's mother, but he did have another surprise for Gail. Gail had an identical twin sister who had been adopted by another family in the same state. "Wow! How incredibly exciting! I can't wait to meet her." Within two days Gail had contacted her twin sister whose name was Amy. Amy didn't know about Gail either. They were both really excited to meet and set a lunch date in a nearby town.

Gail could barely contain her excitement and nervousness as she drove to meet her sister. "Wow! I have an identical twin sister," she said aloud and wondered how much they had in common. She lit a cigarette in the car to try to take the edge off her nervousness.

At the restaurant, she recognized Amy immediately. They were exactly the same height, had exactly the same hair and the same eyes. There was just one major difference between them physically. Amy weighed about 100 pounds less than Gail! "Wow! You're beautiful," Gail said as she hugged Amy.

Lunch went really well. The sisters clicked and talked incessantly about their respective families and upbringing. Amy, a graduate student majoring in health and a part-time yoga instructor, ordered a vegetable salad wrap, Gail had her usual – a cheeseburger with a side of onion rings. After they got comfortable with one another, Gail shared her breast cancer experience with Amy. "Oh, I'm so sorry to hear that," Amy said sympathetically.

"Well, how did you handle your breast cancer?" Gail asked.

"What do you mean?" Amy responded questioningly.

"Your breast cancer. How did you deal with it? Did you undergo radiation, surgery, or what?"

"I've never had breast cancer," Amy said with a rather surprised look on her face.

"What do you mean you've never had breast cancer? We're identical twins. We have the exact same genetic makeup! How could you not have had breast cancer if I've had breast cancer?"

"I don't understand. Why would I have developed breast cancer?"

"Because we're twins, and breast cancer is genetic."

"I don't believe that. Who told you that?"

"Everybody knows breast cancer is genetic!"

"Gail, I may have the same breast cancer gene you do, but that doesn't mean I'm going to get breast cancer. Look, Gail, I don't mean to be rude. I know we're just getting to know each other and I hope we can continue to see each other but did you ever think the reason why you may have *grown* breast cancer, and I did not, is because you are so overweight? You've also smoked four cigarettes during lunch, so far. Do you think your breast cancer may have had something to do with that, too?

This is a fictitious story. I completely made it up. However, I think it is a fairly accurate representation of the way many people think (or don't think) about health. So many people and doctors think a family history of a disease is evidence of a genetic cause for a disease. It rarely occurs to people or doctors that maybe, just maybe, it isn't genetics alone causing diseases like cancer, diabetes, and heart disease, but the choices we make and the environment we live in.

People who grow up and live in the same household together often share similar lifestyles. They have similar habits and values about the foods they choose to eat, the amount of sleep they *choose* to get, the amount of exercise they choose to engage in, and the amount of stress they *choose* to incur in daily life.

Even though Gail was adopted and bore no genetic link to her mother, her aunt, or her grandmother, she was raised in a household that clearly didn't value health. All three ladies had the same body type (except Gail was taller). They were all overweight and they all smoked.

The Honesty Diet

It is very likely Gail ate the same kinds and amounts of foods her mother and her aunt ate thus accounting for her weight. It is also unlikely any of them valued exercise. They all valued stress reduction, but chose to practice their value by smoking cigarettes instead of choosing a healthier practice.

Gail developed breast cancer, not because of her genes, but because of her choices, her habits, and the lifestyle she grew up with. Gail's breast cancer was not genetically passed to her. It was the result of her copying the same unhealthy behaviors her family practiced. Gail chose to live her young adult life at a very low level of health awareness. For her, it was a disease of choice, albeit a largely subconscious choice. So, it is important not to jump the gun, and not make assumptions. Just because a disease "runs in families" is not necessarily an indication the disease is "genetic."

Take Control and Think

I have used prostate and breast cancer as examples for illustrating points raised in this chapter. However, it should be clear I just as easily could have used colon cancer, lung cancer, or any other cancer. Overwhelmingly, cancer is the cumulative, long-term product of your daily choices, both conscious and subconscious. Don't choose to believe your particular cancer is a genetic one or is the result of some unknown environmental toxin. Most likely, it isn't. Stop thinking you are the exception to the rule. Most likely, you aren't. Even if you have a genetic predisposition to a certain kind of cancer, and even if there is a history of a particular cancer in your family, that does not necessarily mean you will grow that cancer. As we discussed in the chapter on genetics, it's largely your choices that determine which genes will be expressed and which will not.

At the risk of being excessively redundant, let me reiterate that if you blame your cancer on a virus or something else *outside* of your control, you give up your control to cancer. You become a victim – a victim who can't change their circumstances. However, when you recognize your *choices* created your level of health, you then have the ability to recognize new choices – different choices – from today forward, which can help you to heal yourself.

~ Section Three ~

Practicing The Honesty Diet™

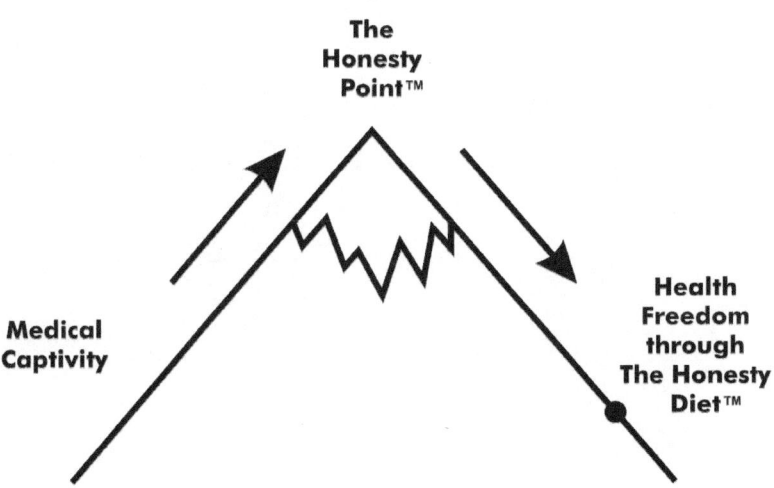

~ 19 ~

INTRODUCTION TO
THE HONESTY DIET™

*You are not overweight
because you are full of fat.*

*You are overweight
because you are full of shit!*

It is now time for us to leave The Honesty Point, begin heading down our intellectual mountain, and start putting what we have learned into action. From now on, you will notice a distinct, less polite change in my tone. This is quite deliberate. In order to put The Honesty Diet into practice *honest* language must be used, which will entail more emotionally-charged and more visceral language with fewer language lies and less political correctness. I know honesty sometimes hurts, especially when we are so out of practice being honest with ourselves but please

The Honesty Diet

be assured, my intent is to be as helpful to you as possible, not to be offensive.

What Is The Honesty Diet?

You may be asking why I've waited until this far into the book to actually get to the "diet" itself. I didn't. The entire book is the diet. However, this diet is so radically different in concept and in practice from any other diet you've ever heard about, you may not have realized you have been learning The Honesty Diet all along. Most diets ultimately boil down to a list or system of foods people should or shouldn't eat. But guess what? We're still sick and we're still fat! In fact, statistics show, we are fatter and sicker than ever! Doing the same thing over and over again and expecting a different result is Einstein's definition of insanity, right? So, why would we once again place all our hopes in yet another list or system of foods you should or shouldn't eat?

Honesty is the key to being healthy and the key to losing weight. In fact, *honesty* is the critical element currently missing from the U.S. healthcare system. It sounds overly simplistic, but honesty is all you really need to succeed. However, like anything else, honesty takes practice.

The Honesty Diet is exactly as it sounds. It is a mental *and* physical "diet" made of honesty, awareness, and thinking. The Honesty Diet is tremendously empowering. If practiced, it provides all you need to accomplish and achieve your health objectives, whether simply to lose weight, get out of pain, or become a more vibrant, healthy person. If practiced, The Honesty Diet can further raise your awareness about your health, longevity, and success in reaching any of your goals.

Everything you need is within you, *if you'll just practice being honest*. It sounds simple, but that's because it is simple. However, due to the plague of medical captivity, with which most of us have been raised and have become accustomed to, this simple concept can be a real challenge.

When practicing The Honesty Diet, you must recognize the reality that a "diet" isn't a temporary way of eating, but a *permanent* way of eating. It is a "healthy eating" and "healthy living" lifestyle, if you will. If you are being honest with yourself, you will recognize there is no such thing as a short-term diet. Diets don't "work" because diets are temporary. Temporary actions produce temporary results.

All Diets Work

Having just stated that diets don't work, allow me now to make a seemingly contradictory statement – All diets work. Yes, you read that correctly. All diets work. All diets work… in *some* people. However, they do not work for the reason you might think they do. They do not work because of a magical formula or special combination of unique kinds of foods. So, the question then is why? *Why* do diets work for *some* people but not for others? What is it those who succeed in any given diet have that those on the exact same diet who fail do not have? We must stop asking ourselves how all these diets differ from one another, and start asking what *all* these diets have in common with one another. The common element is certainly is not what they tell you to eat! After all, some say to eat fat, while other say don't. Some say don't eat carbohydrates, while others say do. Some say to combine certain foods. Others say don't ever combine certain foods with one another. How, then, can *all* diets work?

There are hundreds, perhaps thousands of different kinds of religions in the world. Some are quite similar to one another. Others are quite different. But, the common denominator of all religions is faith. Similarly, all diets have a common denominator as well. Don't worry. I'm not going to suggest it's faith. It's *awareness*. Awareness determines the success or failure of any diet.

In order for a diet to "work" you must "pay attention" to what you are eating and follow the system of the diet with an acute mental awareness. If you maintain a casual awareness when following a diet, you will reap casual or less-than-casual results. On the other hand, if you maintain a focused awareness when following a diet system, you will get focused results, usually the results you seek.

It is less important *which* diet system you follow than it is to simply follow a system… *any* system. That is not to say some diets are not better than others – some are. Some diets are just plain stupid or even dangerous. However, all diets work in some people, but that has very little to do with the specifics of the diet itself and more to do with the person's focus and acute mental awareness toward *following* the diet – *following* the system.

Paying Attention

It isn't *the system* itself that creates positive results, it is *the paying attention to* and *the following of* the system that causes weight loss. When someone follows a diet system, they must assume a heightened awareness about which foods they are eating. The primary cause of weight gain is a lack of awareness, of not paying attention to what you are choosing to eat.

We discussed in an earlier chapter, the Observer Effect. The principle states that the mere observation of an event can *change* the outcome of the event itself. Similarly, simply by being aware of what you are eating – what you are putting into your body – will improve your results. If you want to lose weight, you must *pay attention* to what you are eating. It isn't necessarily the specific foods of a diet plan that cause weight loss, but the individual's consciousness and desire to pay attention to the things he or she chooses to put in their body. Selecting the right kind of diet will improve results, but which diet you select is less important than the mental state, the level of consciousness, the state of awareness you put yourself in while following a diet system.

However, remember that whichever diet you select should be based on honesty. For instance, selecting a popular diet recommending you eat lots of greasy foods and eliminate all foods belonging to a particular energy source, like carbohydrates, wouldn't be an *honest* choice for you. Carbohydrates are probably the most naturally abundant, consumable source of energy on the planet. Does eliminating an entire energy source of food *honestly* sound intelligent to you? If it does, I would strongly suggest you reevaluate your level of honesty. Ask yourself, "Do I really believe this to be true? Or do I just *want to believe* a particular popular diet is healthy because it is a diet allowing me to perpetuate my current addictions?"

The Real Reason Why People Gain Weight

Most people gain weight because they don't pay attention *on a daily basis* to what they are eating. If you are being honest with yourself, you probably already know this to be true. For example, ladies, have you ever tried to lose weight before a special event like a wedding, a Caribbean vacation, or just because summer was just around the corner? Men do this too sometimes, like when trying to get in shape before a sport's season, a job interview, or even before a high school reunion. Often people accomplish their goal. Why is that? First and foremost it is because they *want* to… they *really* want to lose weight. There is an emotional, compelling reason for achieving the weight loss. What is your emotionally-compelling reason? If you don't have one, you probably won't ever lose the weight.

Second, they have focused their attention and awareness on achieving that goal by a specific deadline. But, *honestly*, you already know this, too, don't you? You are already well aware you don't gain thirty, forty, or fifty pounds overnight. So how did you find yourself in such a situation? Weren't you with your body the entire six or twelve months it took to gain the weight? You gained those pounds by not caring or not *paying attention* to your health – to your body – for long, extended periods of time. That is the *only* reason you gained weight.

People who are fit year round are fit because they're *consistently aware* of what they are putting into their bodies. People who are fat year round are that way because they're *consistently unaware* of what they are putting into their bodies. Fit people also intuitively understand the more garbage they eat, the more exercise they need to burn it off. People who are always fit *want* to look fit throughout the year. Because they want it, they achieve it. The problem is most people don't really *want* to be fit and slim, they only *wish* they were.

"Wish" vs. "Want"

One of the reasons so many Americans are fat is because they don't understand the difference between *wishes* and *wants*. Most people say they want to be thin. But, more often than not, that is a lie they tell themselves. They do not *want* to be thin; they only *wish* they were thin. Wish means you'd like to have or be something as long as you don't have to do anything in order to accomplish it. A wish is something a genie gives you after you free him from a magic lamp. A *want*, on the other hand, is something you intend to achieve by setting a *specific* goal preferably with a reasonable deadline, then *focusing* your *awareness* on its achievement *daily*. Wishes are dreams. Wants are goals. If you want to be fit, healthy, and slim then stop *wishing* for it and start *wanting* it.

I have known so many people who have told me they want to be fit. I then ask them, "What do you mean by fit?"

Invariably, they can never answer me. They have no idea what fit means. And, *that is precisely why they aren't fit! They don't know what fit is!* I then ask them, "Does fit mean to lose twenty pounds of fat? Does fit mean you can slip into a size six dress? Does fit mean you'd be comfortable and proud to take your shirt off at the beach?" Rarely, will someone who only *wishes* to be fit answer these questions. They don't answer because they lack the *courage* to set standards for themselves. They're afraid of setting a goal, a deadline, and implementing a plan for achievement. They're afraid it will be too painful. They're afraid of failure. They don't *want* it, they only *wish* it would magically happen to them. By the way, taking dishonest actions, like switching to diet sodas instead of regular soda, is an example of genie wishing – hoping that feeding their sugar addictions with diet soda will magically make them thin. They may be taking action, but it is *dishonest* action, and deep down they know it is dishonest.

Gaining Weight Is Hard Work

Whenever I'm exploring the validity of any statement, I try to mismatch it. That is, I will often reverse the scenario to determine if the statement still holds true. If it doesn't hold up in the mismatch scenario, the statement is often false. For example, let's say instead of trying to *lose* weight, a person wants to *gain* weight. Perhaps he is a bodybuilder or a wrestler who wants to move up in weight class. How can he gain a certain amount of weight, say, twenty pounds, by a certain date? Do you think it is just going to happen to him magically? Not likely. In fact, many people consistently try to gain weight and struggle to do so. Only by putting attention and awareness on what he is eating and how he is exercising on a *daily* basis will that person succeed in gaining the desired weight. Losing weight is no different.

Gaining weight or losing weight isn't something that just happens to us. Both take focus, work, and energy. You don't gain weight suddenly. Usually you must spend a great deal of time and effort making *a lot* of really bad decisions on a *daily* basis for a long period of time in order to gain weight. You must really focus on *not* paying attention to your life and your health. Gaining weight really is, indeed, hard work. However, some of us have become so proficient at gaining weight it almost seems effortless to do so. But, I assure you it isn't. Gaining weight requires just as much effort and energy as does losing weight. It's just you may be out of the habit of losing weight and, instead, have made gaining weight a habit or maybe even an addiction. The same holds true for losing weight. You can't just wish it to happen. Losing weight requires *daily* consciousness – a constant, acute awareness and desire. Fortunately, awareness and desire are free.

Being fat is caused by:

1. Not caring about being fat
   (i.e. "wishing" not wanting to be thin)
   and
2. Not paying attention to what you
   are choosing to eat

That's it. That, in a nutshell, explains the overwhelming majority of cases of being fat. You either choose not to care or you choose not to pay attention. In most cases, the answer is both. That is, you choose not to pay attention *because* you don't care about being fat.

Yeah, but: That isn't always true! I gain weight because I have a bad thyroid and a slow metabolism!

Many people love to blame their weight gain on a dysfunctional thyroid gland and/or a slow metabolism. However, this scenario isn't so different from blaming obesity on one's genetics. Both are equally false. After all, most people don't even know what metabolism is, where their thyroid gland is located, or what either does. The real issue here is why? *Why* do you have a slow metabolism? *Why* do you have a "bad" thyroid? Thyroids don't just suddenly "go bad" for no reason. A more honest assessment would be to ask *why* the thyroid is not functioning properly. Or, *why* is my metabolism so slow? In the overwhelming majority of cases, a slow metabolism is a product of a poor diet, inadequate exercise, a lack of lean muscle mass and even chronic stress.

Thyroid dysfunction is, overwhelmingly, a *product* of long-term dietary neglect and an improper lifestyle, not a *cause* of obesity. An improperly functioning thyroid may exacerbate obesity, but it doesn't *cause* it. An improperly functioning thyroid is frequently a *symptom* of a long-standing nutritional problem. Often, an improperly functioning thyroid and a slow metabolism are the results of a chronically-stressed adrenal system. Chronic adrenal stress is usually caused by a combination of poor diet, poor sleep, little or no exercise, and inadequate stress management.

~ 20 ~

POWER, CONTROL & CHOICES

Which Kind of Person Are You?

There are basically only two kinds of people in the world. There are those who take responsibility, who take control of their lives and thereby become empowered, and there are those who don't. Those who don't take responsibility and control of their lives inevitably place that control in someone else's hands. When you lack control of your own life, when you fail to take responsibility, you give away your power. Without power, you cannot be educated, you cannot be knowledgeable, and you lose your capacity to *think*. This is especially true within a context of health. Unfortunately, more often than not, when you give away your power (by refusing to assume it), you also lose your capacity to be *honest*.

In general, people who are healthy are so because they *assume* their power. They take control of and take responsibility for their health. They make decisions about their health based on education, awareness, thinking, and above all honesty. Similarly, in general, those people who are fat-sick are those who choose to forfeit their power and their control to others. They give in to the medical captivity keeping them sick. Giving away your power may manifest as blindly trusting what a doctor or other health professional tells you instead of researching a health topic for yourself. Or, giving away your power may take the form of blaming your genetics or your occupation for your current health problems.

Which of these two kinds of people are you? If you're not sure, try asking yourself the following questions and, of course, really try to be honest:

- Do you think it's a doctor's job to keep you healthy?
- Do you run to the doctor every time you're sick?
- Do you think disease is something that randomly happens *to* you?
- Do you only think about your health when you are in pain or sick?
- Do you believe medications "fix" health problems?
- Do you think it is unfair you should have to change your lifestyle to be healthy?
- Do you think health care should be free?
- Do you think the government wouldn't allow edible products in the market if not safe?

If you answered "yes" to *any* of these questions, then you may be the kind of person who tends to shun responsibility and relinquish control of your health to others. Let's go through each of these questions and explain why.

Do you think it's a doctor's job to keep you healthy?

Today, many people live their lives with the attitude that they can do as they wish with their bodies and when it breaks down it's a doctor's job to fix it. It is an arrogant sense of entitlement that harms our health and accounts for why so many Americans are fat-sick. This entitlement mentality is also a consequence of the medical captivity people have been conditioned to accept in our society. It is a doctor's job to assist you in *maintaining* your health, not to be responsible *for* your health. People who think it's a doctor's job to be responsible for their health are more often than not fat-sick.

Do you run to the doctor every time you're sick?

Many people rush off to a doctor's office every single time they have the slightest sniffle. They believe a bacteria or virus has pounced upon them and they require medication immediately. Rarely do people ever *think* about what has been going on recently in their lives and how they might be able to address the so-called illness on their own. Rarely will people say something like, "I haven't really made an effort to get to bed at a decent hour recently. Maybe that's why I have a cold now." Or, "Maybe if I didn't drink so much alcohol and eat fast-food all the time, I wouldn't feel so lousy in the morning." Or, "Maybe if I would exercise more and lose some weight, I wouldn't be so depressed all the time." Instead, they automatically call a doctor and expect him or her to "fix" whatever ails them with the latest, expensive (and no doubt side effect-ridden) pharmaceutical drug or herbal supplement. More often than not, people who think like this are fat-sick. They shun responsibility for their own health and place responsibility onto others. Rarely will they recognize that it is the *way they think* (or don't think) that makes them unhealthy.

Do you think disease is something that randomly happens *to* you?

People always act surprised when they find out they have something like colon cancer or heart disease. Sometimes, they even say things like, "How could I have colon cancer? I was fine last year at my annual physical." People frequently believe they "catch" a cold or they "catch" cancer. Healthy-thinking people understand that disease almost always develops *only* in susceptible individuals. What makes a person susceptible or not isn't their genetics but the *daily* decisions they make.

Do you only think about your health when you are sick or in pain?

Unhealthy-thinking people only think about their health when they are sick or in pain. Interestingly, it is this ignorance that makes them unhealthy in the first place. Healthy-thinking people, on the other hand, think about their health *daily*. That is why they exercise, eat well, sleep well, and relax on a *daily* basis. They do these things because *they understand it is those very things which keep them healthy*. Healthy-thinking people rarely need medications. Unhealthy-thinking people usually only start exercising, dieting, or taking supplements *after* they have become sick. They only think about health *after* they have already lost it. They don't recognize they have to focus on their health *daily* in order to keep it.

Do you believe medications "fix" health problems?

Unhealthy-thinking people believe medications "fix" health problems. Healthy-thinking people understand that medications, in general, "cover up" the real problem and often cause more problems. Healthy-thinking people understand a need for medication means there is something wrong with how they are living. Healthy-thinking people understand if they need a medication, most likely they really just have to change something about their lives in order to stay off the medication.

For a healthy-thinking person, the need for an antidepressant often means a person doesn't eat properly and doesn't exercise. A need for blood pressure medication often means a person doesn't eat well and is overweight. A need for sleep medication often means the person doesn't create for himself or herself an environment conducive to rewarding sleep. A need for pain medication often means a person abuses their body and eats garbage foods that cause inflammation and premature degeneration. Healthy-thinking people recognize that if medications "fixed" health problems our country's citizens would be healthy by now. Unhealthy-thinking people don't think about things like this, because unhealthy-thinking people don't generally *think* at all. People who think medications fix health problems usually take a lot of medication, yet they still aren't healthy! Does that *really* sound intelligent to you?

Do you think it is unfair you should have to change your lifestyle in order to be healthy?

Healthy-thinking people understand if they're having a health problem, it is likely something they are doing that is causing the problem, *and they are willing* to modify that behavior. Unhealthy-thinking people are stubborn. They refuse to recognize how their daily decisions adversely affect their health. They'd rather take medications so they don't think they'll have to change their behavior or break their addictions.

Unhealthy-thinking people drink soda and then wonder why they develop osteoporosis (many carbonated beverages are understood to contribute to bone loss). Unhealthy-thinking people eat junk foods that contain toxins like trans-fats and then wonder why they are so fat. Unhealthy-thinking people eat sugar excessively for years and then say "diabetes runs in my family," erroneously blaming their diabetes on faulty genetics. People who think it is unfair they should have to change their lifestyle for health reasons shun responsibility for their health. They have no power – and that is precisely why they are fat-sick.

Do you think health care should be free?

This is a big one. In general, people who think health care should be free in this country tend to shun responsibility for their own health. I know many people feel medical care is enormously expensive. However, one of the things keeping Americans as healthy as they are currently (which, of course, isn't saying very much) is the expense associated with medical care.

I hope health care *never* becomes free in this country. If it does, it will be perceived as a "get out of jail free" card for everybody. If health care becomes free there will no longer be an incentive for people to take care of themselves. Why should they? *They* won't have to pay for treatment if and when they get sick. "Free health care" is an increasingly popular political language lie in the United States. What "free health care" really means, however, is "I shouldn't ever have to think about my health or bother with maintaining my health." It is another arrogant entitlement mentality. Yet, it is this very attitude – this "gimme" attitude – that has made us such a fat-sick country.

Don't Take Advice From Fat Doctors!

Do you think the government wouldn't allow edible products in the market if not safe?

Healthy-thinking people are able to look around, *think*, and see the problem with this belief. A healthy-thinking person has a robust skepticism about what they are told is and isn't healthy. For example, I personally do not think our current government food organizations have our best health interests in mind. I contend money, not ethics and honesty, run these groups. I do not trust these organizations. When they say a food substance is safe, I never take their word for it. I do my own honest investigation and run my findings through my own honesty-thinking algorithms before deciding if it is something I should put in my body. *I'm* the one who decides whether it is safe for me, not *them*. I have control. I have the power.

Most people simply presume if the government says something is generally regarded as safe (GRAS), then it must have been tested. However, that is not the standard operating procedure of most government organizations. Most consumable items are not tested for safety before being made available to the public (unless it is a drug). In general, consumable goods are assumed to be safe until proven otherwise.

Each year drugs are removed from pharmacy shelves for causing death or harmful, devastating side effects. Obviously these drugs weren't safe, yet, they were approved by government agencies. Healthy-thinking people pay attention to and act upon news stories detailing the incestuous relationship government food and drug-

The Honesty Diet

regulating agencies have with food and pharmaceutical manufacturers. Healthy-thinking people pay attention to news stories about faked and "doctored" medical studies that had earlier "proven" a drug to be safe. In the world of food, money talks and health walks. It is my opinion trans-fats, sugar substitutes, and other food additives enter the marketplace each year, not necessarily because they are safe, but because they are profitable.

Unhealthy-thinking people bask in their ignorance, believing if something weren't safe, the government wouldn't allow it on the market. Unhealthy-thinking people simply trust these government and/or medical groups. Not surprisingly, those I know who trust these groups tend to be unhealthy people. They also, more often than not, tend to be heavy people. Coincidence? I doubt it. They relinquished their power to others with different interests and objectives than their own, then wonder why they are fat-sick. Healthy-thinking people assume their power and make their own decisions. Unhealthy-thinking people relinquish their power and allow others to make decisions for them.

If after doing this exercise, you have discovered you tend to be one of those people who shun responsibility for their health, that's OK. You can easily become one of the responsible ones. You can become a healthy-thinking person. All you have to do is *decide*. Reclaim your control – assume your power. Decide it is *your* job and no one else's to be responsible for your health. In fact, doing so is the honest thing to do. Anything less is simply delusional. If you say you don't have time to be that kind of person,

Don't Take Advice From Fat Doctors!

recognize that as just another language lie. You do have time. You just don't *value* your health.

The following beliefs or ways of thinking are examples illustrating the difference in thought between healthy-thinking people and unhealthy-thinking people – between those people who *take* responsibility for their health and those who *shun* responsibility for their health.

Unhealthy-thinking People:
"If I need a drug, it will make me healthy."

Healthy-thinking People:
"If I'm considering a drug, there's something in my life I need to change."

Unhealthy-thinking People:
"If I have high blood pressure, it must be genetic."

Healthy-thinking People:
"If my blood pressure seems high, it must be caused by something I am doing."

The Honesty Diet

> Unhealthy-thinking People:
> *"If I have depression, a drug will fix it."*
>
> Healthy-thinking People:
> *"If I feel depressed, I must not be eating properly, sleeping properly, getting enough sunlight and/or getting enough exercise."*

> Unhealthy-thinking People:
> *Pay doctors to take an interest in their health*
>
> Healthy-thinking People:
> *Take an interest in their own health and pay doctors for assistance*

> Unhealthy-thinking People:
> *See the need for drugs as the <u>end</u> of their health problems*
>
> Healthy-thinking People:
> *See the consideration of drugs as a sign they should <u>begin</u> to address the <u>real</u> problem*

> Unhealthy-thinking People:
> *Say, "How do I get this drug?" (i.e. government assistance, insurance, generic, etc.)*
>
> Healthy-thinking People:
> *Say, "How do I get off this drug!"*

These beliefs reflect a person's style of thinking about their health – one of empowerment and control, or one of victimization. They're meant to be examples only. They are not necessarily complete under each and every circumstance. For example, healthy-thinking people often use doctors, too. However, they don't subordinate their health interest or their control to their doctors.

Reassume Your Power

Each day, Americans are deciding to be healthy or to be sick – to be fit or fat – to be responsible for their health, or to not be responsible for their health. If you want to be healthy you simply must assume your power, and you must take responsibility for and control of your health and your life. *The way to initiate this process is to practice being honest.* You must stop blaming things outside yourself for your health problems.

You are not fat because you don't have time to exercise. You are fat because you don't *value* exercise and therefore you don't *make* the time for exercise. You are not sick because your boss is working you too hard. You are sick because you *choose* not to take care of yourself (taking care of yourself may require finding another job). You are not tired because of your children. You are tired because you do not *value* rest and because you do not exercise. You are not sick because of a bacterial infection. You are sick because you chose not to take care of your body, which then made you *susceptible* to that bacterium. You are not sick because your health insurance doesn't cover all the drugs you've been told you need. You are sick because you *choose* not to do the things that would keep you from needing the drugs in the first place. Sickness isn't something that happens to you. In the overwhelming majority of cases, it is something you *choose*.

Although I belong to no religion, I have always liked the quote "God helps those who help themselves." Stop waiting for someone else to save you and, instead, help yourself. Stop believing your government or your employer owes you something. Stop believing things happen *to* you instead of *by* you. Everything you need to be healthy is within you right now, right this second! But if you want to unlock that magic you're going to need the right key, which is rarely found in a drug; and it's almost never surgery. The key to your health lies within your ability to communicate *honestly* with yourself. Value yourself, get selfish, and put yourself first!

The truth of the matter is most people don't *want* to think about their health. They relinquish their power of thinking to others, like doctors or even the authors of health books – like this one. They just want a list or a system detailing foods they should eat and foods they shouldn't eat – anything that will not require thinking!

But the truth is I can't give you such a list, and even if I could I wouldn't because it would rob you of what you need to be healthy... your capacity to think. However, I can give you the next best thing. I can teach you the ability to *think* about the foods you *choose* to make your body out of and I can give you methodologies to help make these decisions easier for you. You will not believe how easy it is to be fit and healthy if you will just reclaim your inborn ability to *think* and be *honest*! Remember: Healthy people think. Unhealthy people do not think. If you are not healthy, it's probably because you're either not *thinking* or you don't *want* to be healthy!

~ 21 ~

BELIEFS WITHOUT THOUGHT

Beliefs Without Thought

The quality of your health and of your diet is largely a function of your beliefs about what a healthy food is and what is not. Some people are terrified about eating eggs and avocados because they *believe* cholesterol is evil. Other people believe sugar is bad and *believe* artificial sugar substitutes are healthy. Still others *believe* salt is bad because they *believe* salt is the reason for their high blood pressure. So they choose to use artificial salt substitutes *believing* they are making a healthier choice. Some people avoid eating fat because they *believe* fat makes them fat. I have emphasized the word *believe* in the preceding sentences for a specific reason. I say *believe* instead of *think*, because, for the most part, there is very little *thinking* actually going on in these people's minds.

While these people *believe* something is good or bad for them, if you ask them simple questions about the things they believe such as, "Why do you believe cholesterol is bad for you? Can you even tell me what the biological function of cholesterol is?" Or, "Do you *really* think your body is making cholesterol by mistake?" Overwhelmingly, they can't answer these questions. That is because these people generally only have *beliefs*, not *thoughts*. They do not necessarily know or understand why they believe the things they do. For example, I eat eggs and avocados several times each week because I *understand* (through personal research and *thinking*) that these are healthy foods. Many others *believe* these foods are dangerous, but they don't know why they *believe* that. In this section we are going to deconstruct some popular, yet erroneous *beliefs* about certain types of food substances and see whether or not these beliefs actually make any sense.

Sugar Substitutes Are Not Healthy

One of the biggest beliefs out there is that consuming sugar causes obesity and diabetes. This isn't true. But if it were, would that mean consuming a sugar substitute is healthier? I hope you answered no. It could easily and convincingly be argued that eating synthetic sugar substitutes is far less healthy than eating a normal, natural substance like sugar. It is not the *consumption* of sugar that causes obesity and diabetes. It is the *excessive* consumption of sugar that can cause these health problems. In my opinion, sugar is, dare I say, a "healthy" food source. Our brains and many other parts of our bodies run on sugar. The problem is the *excessive indulgence*, not the sugar itself! Blaming our obesity and diabetes on sugar is a dishonest way of perceiving the problem. People choose to consume excessive sugar in coffee, in candy, in soft drinks and in most processed foods.

For decades, people in the United States have been socially conditioned by so-called "health" marketers to *believe* sugar is evil and, therefore, their synthetic sugar substitute is a healthy alternative. I disagree. Let's say you consume, on average, 500 grams of sugar per day. This is a ridiculous amount of sugar and would be approximately the equivalent of twenty sodas! Clearly, if you were to consume this much sugar you would have overindulged. Under the *belief* that sugar substitutes are a healthy alternative to sugar, do you think it would be healthier to "substitute" those 500 grams of sugar for 500 grams of sugar substitute? I should hope not! Overindulgence is *your* fault, not the sugar's fault. Don't blame the sugar and don't blame the food manufacturer. You *choose* to put excessive amounts of sugar in your body.

If I were forced to make a choice between having to eat real sugar or sugar substitute for the rest of my life, I would without a doubt select real sugar. Sugar is natural. Many sugar substitutes are synthetic. My body was designed to consume and metabolize sugar. My body was not designed to metabolize synthetic substances. Sugar has *never* been pulled off the market for causing cancer and brain tumors. Conversely, sugar substitutes are regularly pulled off the market for causing all sorts of health problems. I know most of us have read, at one time or another, the infinitesimally small-font warning on the side of a certain packaged sugar substitute reading something to the effect of: "Warning: This product has been known to cause cancer in lab animals." Have you ever seen a cancer warning on a package of real sugar? No? Then why do so many people think sugar substitutes are healthier than eating natural sugar? Where did this belief come from?

If you're being honest with yourself, the new awareness, then, is:

Don't put things in your body it wasn't designed to break down.

You don't put diesel fuel in an unleaded car. So don't put substances like sugar substitutes in your body. Your body wasn't designed for it. Do you really think if you completely exchanged sugar for synthetic sugar substitute in your diet you would prevent obesity and diabetes? Honestly, does that *really* make sense to you? If it does, I would like to sell you oceanfront property in Colorado.

Only Fat People Drink Diet Soft Drinks

Maybe it's just me, but the only people I ever see drinking diet soft drinks containing artificial sugar are fat-sick people. Why do you think that is? I think it's because most fat-sick people have a *belief system* about health which makes them and keeps them fat. Part of that belief system is that diet soda is healthier than regular soda. Some people even believe there is a special ingredient in diet soda helping them to lose weight! Now, if we are being

The Honesty Diet

honest, we know neither diet soda, nor regular soda is healthy. But to suggest diet soda is *healthier* than regular soda because the diet soda contains a sugar alternative is just ridiculous.

I don't drink soda. Soda is probably the second least healthy edible "thing" or "substance" available today, second only to edible "things" containing trans-fats. However, if I were forced to select between drinking regular soda or diet soda, you bet I would pick the *regular* soda. I would select regular soda because sugar is a natural, normal food substance my body can safely and easily break down.

Now, I know some people would argue the sugar found in most kinds of soda is something called high-fructose corn syrup (or HFCS) and isn't really raw or natural sugar. I agree. High fructose corn syrup, like that commonly found in many soft drinks, wreaks havoc on the body, particularly your pancreas and immune system. However, in my opinion, it is still less damaging than sugar substitutes – some of which were pulled off the market for being suspected of causing brain tumors in animals and suspected of causing disease in humans.

Again, *real* sugar has never been pulled off the market because it's a safe, natural food source! Don't be afraid of sugar. Be afraid of your gluttony. It is your *choice* to over-consume. You choose to buy the jumbo-size drinks. It's self-inflicted injury due to our cultural *addiction* to sugar. Stop trying to blame your health problems on things outside of yourself. The enemy is within.

Addiction Revisited

Why do some people crave sugar and others do not? Contrary to what your doctor or news media outlet may have told you, I don't think it has anything to do with your genetics. It has to do with addiction. Many years ago, I had a fierce addiction to sugar. I was an addict, a junkie. But, I broke that addiction once I reached my Honesty Point about sugar and recognized the negative effects its excessiveness was having on my life. Today, I don't crave candy, soft drinks or coffee.

Sugar addiction, the chronic, excessive consumption of sugar, is the second most prevalent form of substance abuse in the United States. We tend to think of things like heroin use or alcoholism when we use the word addiction. However, far more people die each year from sugar addiction in the form of diabetes, cancer, and heart disease than from alcoholism and heroin *combined*.

At the time of this writing, annual deaths from alcoholism in the United States are somewhere around 20,000. Deaths from all illegal drug use are somewhere around 25,000 per year. These two statistics total 45,000 deaths per year. However, deaths from diabetes alone number around 75,000 deaths per year! There is simply no comparison here. Sugar addiction is second only to tobacco in terms of addiction prevalence (causing death) in the United States. Type II diabetes, a completely *choice*-based disease directly related to obesity, in many cases, comprises about 90% of all diabetes cases and is caused, in part, by chronic, long-term and excessive sugar consumption.

The Honesty Diet

At this point you might say, "Right! I agree. Sugar is bad. That's why I use a sugar substitute." But you don't need a sugar substitute. You need to break your sugar addiction! The only reason you consider using a sugar substitute in the first place is because you're a junkie. Only junkies use sugar substitutes, just as only nicotine addicts use a nicotine patch (a cigarette substitute). The *honest* truth is, you don't *want* to stop using sugar, even though you know you should. Your desire for a sugar substitute is based upon intuitively knowing you *should* stop excessively consuming sugar. Your seeking out of a sugar substitute without having to give up the daily "high" you get from sugar is evidence of an inner conflict you are having in your mind. You viscerally know your excessive sugar consumption is unhealthy, but instead of breaking your addiction, you are turning to a sugar substitute. That isn't healthy. It's just substituting one vice for another.

We discussed this phenomenon in a slightly different manner earlier in this book. Substituting one thing for another without really changing anything is another version of a language lie. It is equivalent to saying, "I'm not fat. I'm just big boned!" Or, "Oh, I don't use heroin. Heroin is bad. I use crystal meth, instead!" You can say, "Oh, I don't use sugar. Sugar is bad. I use a sugar substitute." But the truth is turning to a sugar substitute is evidence of your addiction, your unwillingness to change, and you are not really wanting to give up the high you get from your sugar addiction. Using sugar substitutes is a *dishonest* way of attempting to convince yourself you're trying to be healthier. But you're not really trying to be healthier! You need to break your addiction, not exchange one unhealthy addiction for another.

Trying to convince a sugar addict of their addiction is often like trying to talk a drunk person out of driving their car home. It rarely can be done. Recognizing oneself as an addict – a junkie – is something a person must *want* to see. If they want to see it they will because they have an *honest* desire to be healthier, to free themselves of their addiction.

In most cases, a person cannot be convinced intellectually by others of their addiction. It must be self-recognized. It is for that reason I cannot "sell you" on the idea that you may be addicted to sugar or something else. You must recognize it yourself, and you must *want* to break the addiction. Self-recognition of one's junkie status requires tremendous *courage* that everyone has but few people assume. Recognition of one's addiction to sugar or anything else produces control. Control leads to the power to break the addiction. The most prominent symptom of addiction is often one's unawareness of it, which is why so many Americans are fat-sick.

Salt Substitutes Are Not Healthy

Salt substitutes are also poor health choices. So-called "health" product marketers and health "experts" have successfully convinced a significant percentage of the U.S. population that salt is the evil culprit behind high blood pressure. In my opinion, nothing could be farther from the truth. All across America, people (particularly those of the baby-boomer generation) are purchasing salt substitutes and replacing their regular table salt with them because they actually *believe* (again, not *think*) this will help lower their blood pressure. As an exercise in *honesty*, let's actually look at the real causes of high blood pressure and how Americans tend to lie to themselves about trying to lower it.

Blood Pressure and Body Fat

A major cause of high blood pressure isn't necessarily the amount of salt you consume, but your body weight, specifically, body fat. The heavier you are, the harder your heart has to pump to circulate blood throughout your body. Many health professionals will tell you excessive body weight is a *contributing factor* to high blood pressure, not a *cause*. Don't believe this. This is a language lie people tell themselves so they won't have to change. Being overweight is a *cause* of, not a *contributing factor to*, high blood pressure.

Sixty-six percent of Americans are fat. This statistic includes "overweight" people. Remember: If we are being honest, "overweight" is just a language lie for "fat." The percentage of Americans with high blood pressure is currently about 33%. I'd be willing to bet most of those with high blood pressure also fall into the 66% category of Americans who are fat. Coincidence? Probably not. Is it intelligent to spend time and energy trying to reduce salt consumption by switching it out for a salt substitute, when the real issue much of the time is weight?

Don't Take Advice From Fat Doctors!

Here is an example of the kind of conversation I have had with people:

"I have high blood pressure, Doc. I don't like taking blood pressure medication. I've been taking an herbal supplement, which seems to have helped a little bit. What else can I do about it?"

"Address the cause," I say.

"What do you mean?" they respond, perplexed.

"Why do you *think* you have high blood pressure?"

"I don't know. Genetics?"

"Go look in the mirror and try to answer that question yourself. Why do you think you have high blood pressure?"

"What are you getting at?"

"You are supposed to have high blood pressure." I reply. "It is the only *intelligent* thing your body could do under its dire circumstances. Look, I don't mean to be rude, but you must be well aware you're overweight. By *choosing* to be overweight, your heart has to work much harder to adequately circulate blood throughout your body. It could easily be argued your body *needs* to have high blood pressure so long as you are going to remain so overweight. You asked me what you can do about it. I told you to address the *cause*. An herbal supplement isn't going to address the *cause*. *Think* about it. Is the reason you have high blood pressure because there isn't enough herbal supplement in your body? Of course, not. The reason you have high blood pressure is because you are fat. Lose the weight and you'll most likely lose the high blood pressure."

"But don't some thin people have high blood pressure, too?"

"Sure. But it's more rare. Don't try to use an exception to divert attention away from the real cause of your problem. The fact of the matter is you are fat and you have high blood pressure because you are fat. Your body is trying to *protect* you. It *has* to raise your blood pressure to adequately circulate blood throughout your body. The healthiest thing to do is lose weight immediately. That way, your body won't have to maintain such high blood pressure."

"I could just keep taking blood pressure medication, can't I?"

"You could. But in my opinion, that would be pretty stupid of you."

"Why would that be stupid?"

"Because your body is *deliberately* raising your blood pressure *for a healthy reason*. Your body knows it *needs* to have higher blood pressure if you are going to continue to be so fat. If you artificially lower your blood pressure with medication, you won't be properly circulating blood throughout your body. Obviously, this is unhealthy. Very likely, it will cause other serious health problems later in your life."

"But if taking blood pressure medication wasn't healthy for me, why would my doctor prescribe it?"

"Sometimes we forget that doctors are people, too, and some of them don't necessarily *think* any more clearly than non-doctors do. Like other professionals, many doctors (not all) just do what they were taught in school or what their pharmaceutical sales representatives tell them to do. In general, doctors try to bring your blood pressure down to a statistical norm, but that effort often assumes everyone's blood pressure should be the same. In my opinion, if you are overweight, you may need to have higher blood pressure. More importantly, you need to lose weight immediately. But if you're not *willing* to do what it takes to lose the weight, you may need to have higher blood pressure in order to be as healthy as you can be while fat. Lose the weight and I think you will find your 'high' blood pressure vanishes."

Obviously, conversations like this one require having a great deal of preexisting rapport with someone before I can speak so honestly with him or her. However, one of the most common responses is, "Wow! I never thought of it that way. It never occurred to me my body may be *deliberately* raising my blood pressure for an intelligent, *healthy* reason." I then explain to them that very few people actually ever *think* about health because for nearly a century we as a society, through medical captivity, have been trained not to think about our health. We have merely been conditioned, like dogs, to respond to perceived authority symbols, like a white coat and stethoscope, and follow standard "health" advice – no matter how *unintelligent* some of that advice may be.

Blood Pressure and Exercise

A second major *cause* of high blood pressure, again, isn't salt consumption, but a lack of exercise. Obviously, this second cause relates directly to being fat. However, it bears further discussion. Exercise helps lower blood pressure even in people who are not overweight by strengthening the heart and vessels, improving overall circulation, and reducing stress. Exercise also helps lower stress and improves poor cholesterol ratios.

Get off your rear and use your body. Your body was designed to move. It was designed to exercise *daily*. It wasn't designed to sit in front of a television or computer screen all day. If you want to have normal, healthy blood pressure you have to exercise daily. So use it or lose it!

House Cleaning Isn't Exercise

While on the subject of exercise, I'd like to talk about another language lie permeating society. It seems almost every week now I read in a magazine or hear on the news of a so-called "health" tip that makes my head shake and eyes roll. For example, one such tip cited a study concluding that typical daily activities like house cleaning burn calories and, therefore, count toward one's daily exercise requirement. This assertion is ridiculous. It implies people may already be exercising enough and just not know it. The premise gives people yet another excuse for not exercising. People can say, "I don't have to go to the gym or go for a walk today. I already exercised when I vacuumed the carpets! That counts as exercise!" Really?

Does that *really* make sense to you? Is that really *honest*? Tell you what: Go look in the mirror, *again*. Are you still fat? If the answer is yes, then normal daily activities like house cleaning don't count as exercise! Otherwise you'd be thin. Stop lying. Your body was designed to exercise daily.

These so-called health articles I come across are part of America's fat problem. Stephen Covey has another well-known quote: "You can't *talk* your way out of a problem you *behaved* yourself into." Yet we keep trying to talk ourselves out of the things we need to do to be fit and healthy. "Health" articles like this one try to convince us we are already exercising enough. But that simply isn't true if 66% of Americans are fat! This is a completely dishonest "health" article. Be *honest*. Go exercise.

Blood Pressure and Alcohol

A third major cause of high blood pressure still isn't salt consumption. It's alcohol consumption. Many health professionals will tell you it's OK to drink alcohol if you have high blood pressure. I think this is terribly irresponsible. We know drinking alcohol increases blood pressure. Let's put on our honesty glasses and examine *why* doctors hesitate to tell people to stop drinking alcohol.

Alcohol Addicts

Telling people to stop drinking alcohol is unpopular. Most health professionals and doctors don't tell their patients to stop drinking alcohol. Instead they say weaker things like, "You can drink alcohol, but do so *in moderation.*" Why do you think that is? Why do they say "in moderation?" It's because so many patients are alcohol addicts!

Patients don't want to hear they have to break their addiction and doctors fear their patients (a.k.a. their customers) might seek out another doctor who will not tell them to stop drinking. Why might patients consider changing doctors? Don't they want to fix their high blood pressure? The honest answer is, no – at least, not if it means giving up their addiction. The truth is many patients are being dishonest with themselves. They aren't really interested in lowering their blood pressure.

Although few people have the courage to say it, alcohol is the number one drug of choice for Americans. Consequently, a high percentage of Americans are alcohol addicts. This does not mean they are *alcoholics*, but they are *alcohol addicts*. Remember: the definition of an addict is one who must do something daily. If you can't function without a daily drink of alcohol, if you don't feel quite right in the evening without at least one drink, if you can't relax at the end of the day without a drink, guess what? You are an alcohol addict.

Think about it, and be honest. What if we replaced the word *alcohol* with the word *cigarette*? Would you consider that person an addict? Let's see. If you can't function without a daily *cigarette*, if you don't feel quite right in

Don't Take Advice From Fat Doctors!

the evening without at least one *cigarette*, if you can't relax at the end of the day without a *cigarette*; would you consider this person an addict? Of course, you would. Why? Because they can't function without that cigarette! We could repeat this exercise with any number of things:

- If you can't function without a daily marijuana joint...
- If you can't function without a daily cup of coffee...
- If you can't function without a daily cola...
- If you can't function without a daily doughnut...

So why should this standard be any different for alcohol? The only honest answer to that question is – *it isn't any different*! It's just alcohol addiction is socially acceptable in the United States because such a high percentage of people in this country are alcohol addicts. Therefore, *alcohol appears innocent only by preponderance*! Think about it. The only reason Prohibition failed in the 1920s and 1930s was because such a high percentage of Americans were already alcohol addicts. Those representatives who repealed the 18th Amendment were alcohol addicts themselves who represented a constituency of alcohol addicts!

What if, instead of alcohol, the number one drug of choice for Americans was cocaine? What if most Americans, at the end of the day, came home from work and instead of pouring themselves a drink, sniffed a line of cocaine? What do you think doctors would say? Do you think doctors would say, "Don't use cocaine. It isn't healthy for you?" I firmly contend that they would *not* say this. In fact, if most Americans did use cocaine regularly,

The Honesty Diet

I'm convinced most doctors would say, "It's OK to use cocaine *in moderation!*" I'm serious. I know it sounds a bit preposterous, but I'm not making a joke. They would say this because if cocaine were as socially acceptable as alcohol is today, most doctors wouldn't dare suggest to patients they should stop using. First of all, doctors would be afraid of losing their patients to another doctor who wouldn't tell patients to stop using cocaine. Second, many doctors would probably be using cocaine daily themselves! We have a tendency to forget that doctors are just people with health problems, weight problems, and substance abuse problems just like so many other people.

The truth is most health professionals don't have the *courage* to tell their addict patients to stop drinking alcohol even though it is a primary cause of their high blood pressure, pain syndrome, or other health problem. People would rather keep their alcohol addiction and just take medication to counteract their addiction's side effects (i.e. high blood pressure), than to stop drinking and get off the prescription drug. The reality is many people who take blood pressure medication take the prescription drug *not* to lower their blood pressure, but to facilitate their alcohol addiction.

This same principle applies to losing weight. Doctors don't tell patients they are fat and need to lose weight, because if they do they will probably lose that person as a patient. Or, they may be sued, reprimanded, or even lose their license to practice! For example, in 2005 the Associated Press news reported a doctor was being reprimanded by his state board and possibly sued by a patient because he, the doctor, had the audacity to inform a patient that she was too fat. According to the report, the patient's *feelings* were hurt by the comment, so she filed a complaint with the state. Similarly, as we have already discussed, many doctors don't tell their patients to stop drinking alcohol or lose weight because they themselves drink alcohol and are overweight! To suggest that to a patient would seem hypocritical and make the doctors feel uncomfortable themselves. You see? The system is set up to perpetuate our addictions and illnesses.

Dehydration and Blood Pressure

We have discussed three major factors that *cause* (not "contribute to") high blood pressure: high body fat, lack of exercise, and alcohol consumption. However, there is another major *cause* of blood pressure issues, and it happens to be, in my opinion, the most important one. No, once again, it is still not salt consumption, but yes, it is related to salt. Now, the exact physiologic mechanisms of blood pressure are complex and too cumbersome for purposes of this philosophical discussion; however, in my opinion, the most important factor causing blood pressure issues is *dehydration*. It isn't necessarily that people consume too much *salt* in their diet (although this can be true). It is people do not have enough *water* in their bodies to properly regulate blood pressure.

At this point, many would say, "But I do drink water constantly! I drink water all day long. I drink so much water that I am sick of it!" That is not what I mean by consuming more water. We shouldn't be "drinking"

The Honesty Diet

more water. We need to "eat" more water. Yes, I said "eat" more water.

Most Americans are *severely* dehydrated. Their *cells* are severely dehydrated. And, contrary to popular belief, you don't hydrate cells by *drinking* water. You hydrate cells by *eating* water. Eating water means eating lots of good ol' fruits and vegetables. Fruits and vegetables are, generally, 60% to 95% water. The more fresh, raw fruits and vegetables you eat, the more you hydrate your cells and the less important a variable like salt becomes in your diet. As a result of hydrating your cells, your blood pressure modulates properly. It is a function of balance, not necessarily trying to eliminate salt from your diet. As we shall soon see, hydration is a major principle of The Honesty Diet. (Please note: I am not referring to the amount of water in your bloodstream. I am referral to the overall amount of water in your entire body. After all, you may be surprised to discover that *drinking* too much water at once can actually *cause* blood pressure problems, as well.)

There is a body of water in the Middle East called the Dead Sea. Its water contains eight times the concentration of salt as the Atlantic Ocean. Three million years ago, the Dead Sea was a part of the Mediterranean Sea. But since then the landmasses shifted so much so that most of the water has left the area. It isn't that The Dead Sea has too much salt in it now, but rather, it doesn't have enough water in it anymore. The concentration of the water in the Dead Sea is so high it cannot support *any* marine life, hence the name the Dead Sea.

The only life form the Dead Sea can support is some types of bacteria. Hmmm? Only *bacteria* can survive in the *Dead* Sea? Is it possible, then, human illnesses, caused by bacteria build up, result from of a lack of water in the body? Is it possible dehydration of the body increases the *relative* concentration of salt in our bodies where bacteria proliferate? Furthermore, it is no wonder most Americans are constipated! They are completely dehydrated and are drying out, just like the Dead Sea. If the Dead Sea were drying up, how would you suggest we fix it? By removing the salt from it? Of course, not. You'd have to add water! The same thing holds true with *your* body of water.

I am not suggesting salt intake is unimportant, but come on people, let's put things in perspective here, shall we? How much salt we consume isn't really that important unless these other four major *causes* of blood pressure problems have been addressed and resolved. Are you thin? Are you exercising? Are you still drinking alcohol? Are you "eating" enough water? Take care of these, first. Then and only then, in my opinion, should salt intake be considered. Don't lie to yourself. Be honest. It will make you much healthier and happier. Trying to lower your blood pressure by substituting salt for fake salt is as useless and foolish as trying to empty the Dead Sea of salt with a tablespoon.

The epitome of dishonesty is that we, the fattest nation on the planet, *pretend* to lower our blood pressure by decreasing the amount of salt we consume, when the real problem is we are fat, sedentary, dehydrated, alcohol-addicted people. Switching to a salt substitute is a useless, pointless gesture. Instead, if you are willing to be honest, if you are willing to demonstrate *courage*, then address the real problem first. If you do, I think you will find you won't have to worry anymore about how much salt you consume.

This book is not specifically about high/low blood pressure or any other specific disease or condition, other than the metaphoric *disease of dishonesty* and the *disease of medical captivity*. I only use blood pressure as one of dozens of possible examples. I just as easily could have deconstructed other sacred medical beliefs, including myths about cholesterol, cancer, osteoporosis, or Alzheimer's disease. This blood pressure example illustrates how people lie to themselves about trying to be healthy, and remember, if you are going to lie to yourself about your health, you forfeit any right to complain about your health. However, as you rediscover how to be honest about your health, you will accumulate great awareness, control, and power toward improving your health.

If you do the mirror test described earlier in this book on a regular basis, you'll be able to take care of many health concerns on your own. *Just be honest*. If you have high blood pressure and you look in the mirror and see a heavy person, don't conclude you have high blood pressure because you eat too much salt! That would be dishonest. If you are fat, and you have high blood pressure, the cause of your high blood pressure is staring you in the face. Be sure to be honest with yourself. Don't decide you aren't *that fat* just because you're not as fat as someone else you know. Don't decide if you are fat or not by comparison or relativity. Decide for yourself, based on your own *honest* standards.

~ 22 ~

PRIORITIES: THE "BIG ROCKS" OF HEALTH

An instructor at a seminar takes out a wide-mouthed jar and begins to place some big rocks into it. After he cannot get any more big rocks into the jar, he then places several smaller rocks into the jar. Next, he pulls out a bag of gravel and begins pouring it into the container. He shakes and sifts the jar until all the gravel has filled the gaps left around the big rocks and the smaller rocks. Then, he pulls out a sack of sand and begins pouring it into the jar. The sand fills the gaps left around the gravel. Lastly, he pulls out a jug of water, pours it into the now dense jar, and screws the cap in place. He then asks his audience, "What was the point of this exercise?" After a few incorrect guesses from the audience, the instructor proclaims: *If you don't put the big rocks in first, they won't fit in later!*

This story illustrates the powerful importance of priorities. When it comes to your health, are you putting your big rocks in first? If you don't, you won't be able to fit them in later either. What are your big rocks? Do you even know? If not, *why*? When it comes to most people's health, everything else in their life comes first: the gravel, the sand, and the water. The big rocks of health never seem to be placed into the jar of life. Is health acquisition and maintenance a priority for you, or and just an afterthought? For most people, it's an afterthought. If you aren't first placing those big rocks in the jar that is your life, you can't act surprised later when you're fat-sick and when your health has failed.

I'm always perplexed by dishonest people who complain about their health and want help. Invariably, I ask them, "What are you doing to improve your health?" To which they usually respond with, "What do you mean?'" You see? Here we go again. We have a person who is living their life at a low level of health awareness. They seem to think health is a given, that it is automatic, that it doesn't require any work, effort, or maintenance on their part. For some reason, they feel *entitled* to good health, regardless of how they may treat themselves. Then later, they wonder why they don't have it. When I tell the "big rocks" story to people and ask them, "What are your big rocks for health?" They usually say things like, "Well, I get an annual physical." As if an annual physical, by itself, actually does anything to *improve* or maintain one's health!

Ask most Americans what their big rocks of health are, and you'll likely get a list of things like prescription drugs, surgery, flu shots, supplements, and health insurance – the things many Americans *believe* produce health. In essence, this is the very reason we are so fat-sick. This is a highly dishonest belief system, one of very low awareness.

We can deduce what the major rules are for being a healthy human being by looking, first and foremost, at what is *required* for a human to survive and thrive. Believe it or not, some of these might surprise you.

The 4 "Big Rocks" of Health

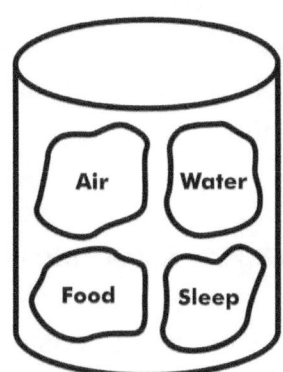

The Honesty Diet is rooted in four big rocks of human health. They are: air, water, sleep and food. Some people add stress reduction as a fifth big rock and still others add spirituality as a sixth. However, in my opinion, these elements are actually *products* of the four big rocks. That is, stress reduction and spirituality *emerge* as a result of proper air, water, sleep, and food.

How many smaller rocks you have in your life is entirely up to you. The important thing is for you to appreciate these four big rocks and to make sure you're putting them in your jar first. They are not trivial. Do not take them for granted. In your life, your big rocks must come *before* career, entertainment, religion, travel, community, *and even family.*

Yeah, but: "That's ridiculous! I can't put my health ahead of my children and family."

Really? Are you sure about that? *Think* about it. Are you an asset or a liability to your children when you are sick? What good are you to your family if you're dead? Without health, things like career, entertainment, and travel really don't have much value.

Big Rock 1: Air (a.k.a. Exercise)

Let's start with the most basic physical human requirement. Can you guess what it is? Many people assume it is food and shelter. That is not the correct answer. The most basic physical human requirement is air. People can survive for quite a while without food. They can go without shelter for even longer periods depending upon numerous conditions. However, humans can only survive three or four minutes without air. Therefore, air is *the single most important* physical requirement for health. However, how common is it for people who wish to improve their health to think about the air they breathe? Many disease conditions are caused by poor air quality. I'm not just talking about hay fever and allergies. I'm talking about things like emphysema and lung cancer. In fact, sound theories exist that all cancers, on some level, involve an oxygen deficiency.

Do you know what your community's air quality is like? Most people do not. I don't like to live in places with poor air quality because I know in the hierarchy of health air quality is paramount. Why? Again, it is because humans can only survive for a few minutes without it. That is why I have multiple air purifiers running in my home 24/7, which help neutralize allergens and pollutants. If you live in a house less than ten years old, the air quality in your house could be worse than the air quality outside due to the off-gassing of home-building materials such as paints, glues, varnishes and carpet fibers. Furthermore, I have a half dozen plants in my bedroom to provide additional oxygen and absorb pollutants and irritants while I sleep. This room is, after all, where I spend one-third of my life!

By the way, did you know poor air quality can make you fat? We have already discussed how chronic stress can cause increases in fat storage. A chronically-heightened sympathetic state of the nervous system sends the rest of your body into a prolonged, panicky survival mechanism known as fight or flight. As a result of this high-stress state, your body thinks there is an ongoing emergency and begins to, rather logically, store fat for survival reasons. Don't you think continuously breathing poor quality air full of carcinogens and other toxins could send your body into a heighten sympathetic state? Can you see how this might contribute to fat storage? So, if humans can only survive for a few minutes without air and if I wish to be a healthy person, I need to choose to live in a place where the air quality is as clean as possible and I must make the air quality in my home as clean and fresh as possible.

In order to determine what places have the best air quality, I use a website call Scorecard: The Pollution Information Site. This site compiles government data which determines air quality, water quality, and other pollution factors by state, county, and postal code. You may want to visit this website and inquire what the pollution is like where you live, work, and play. Depending on what you find and how much you value your health and that of your children, you may subsequently choose to live, work, and play elsewhere.

Directly related to the subject of air and its primary importance in the hierarchy of health is exercise. Many people assume exercise should be its own big rock. However, I consider exercise a part of the air component since exercise is primarily an exerted exchange of air. Exercise is a fundamental requirement for being healthy. If you don't like to exercise, what you are really saying is you don't like being healthy. This attitude will probably harm you throughout your life. Disliking exercise is a choice – a choice which does not serve you. You may want to choose to feel differently about it if you'd like to look better, feel better, be healthier, be wealthier, and have a higher quality of life. I include wealthier because it is very common for someone to work their entire life building a nest egg for retirement, then lose it all treating preventable diseases and cancers. If you choose not to exercise, you are essentially choosing to be fat-sick. If you choose not to exercise you necessarily forfeit your right to complain about your poor health and fat-sick body later.

Exercise is a rule for being human. You can't change this truth. Stop trying to cheat and get around it. Accept it, do it daily, and move forward with your life.

Another reason why air quality is vital to one's health is because of the adverse effects exercise can have on your body if you live in a highly-polluted area. If you live in a highly-polluted area, exercise may actually exacerbate a cancer or other health problem – that is, the more air exchange (exercise) you get of highly toxic, polluted air, the more likely and the sooner you may develop an inhalation-related disease like lung cancer or emphysema. Conversely, the more clean, pollution-free air exchange (exercise) you get, the *less* likely you are to develop such a disease and the higher quality of life you will likely have.

Now, be honest and don't abuse this awareness. You can't justify not exercising because you live in a highly-polluted area. A more honest thought would be maybe you consider living in a place with better air quality so you can exercise more often. And, how often should you exchange air (exercise)? You already know the answer from a previous chapter. If you are committed to your health, it means you exercise daily.

I'm not going to go into detail about exercise. There are already hundreds of books and thousands of online articles on that subject. Just pick activities you like to do… and do them.

The Honesty Diet

Big Rock 2: Water (Hydration)

The second most important physical requirement in the hierarchy of health again, isn't food. It's water. Humans can only survive for a few days or maybe a week at the most without water – either water as a liquid or water from food. Therefore, water is the next most important big rock. Do you know what your community's water quality is? Do you know what carcinogens and other toxins are in your community's water supply? If you drink bottled water, do you really know where that water came from? Several investigations of bottled water were found to be no better than tap water and, in some cases, the bottled water was *worse* than average municipal water.

When people think of consuming water, most people think only about drinking water, but we also *absorb* water from swimming and bathing, and *inhale* water from humidity and shower steam. These additional water sources can be equally contaminated and can cause cancerous conditions in our bodies. The Scorecard website, again, is a great tool for determining the water quality of your community.

I have not one, but two whole-house water filters on my home's water main. I purchase pure, non-chlorinated, non-fluoridated, mineral-rich drinking water from a trusted, frequently-tested source for all my drinking and cooking needs. Furthermore, I ionize my drinking water with an alkalizing water filter and I affix my shower heads with Vitamin C filters to remove any remaining chlorine and chloramines. And, finally, because I live in a semi-arid climate, I sleep with a cool, clean water humidifier in my bedroom to help keep my skin moist. Cumulatively, I almost completely avoid the inhalation or absorption of toxins from public water sources. Municipal water sources often contain toxins, which leach out of the metal and/or plastic pipes used in public infrastructure and residential housing.

Yeah, but: That is not reasonable! I can't move. My job is in this polluted area with polluted air and water. There is nothing I can do about that!

This is not an honest objection. Nobody in this country has a government-dictated job or career. You can move to a cleaner area and get a different job or start a new career if you really wanted to – that is, if you really valued your health. What people with this objection really mean, and can rarely admit, is they value their job or career *more* than they value their health or that of their children. The reason why people fly off the handle when I suggest this is simply because… it's true. The offense they take is *evidence* of the statement's *emotional* charge and its accuracy. If my assertion were not true, it wouldn't cause offense. This is their choice.

There is absolutely nothing wrong with valuing your job more than your health. It is just if you do, admit you have made a choice – a choice with consequences. Your priority may lead to spending most of your hard-earned money from your job treating the cancer or disease your choice produced. It is not uncommon in the United States to have to declare bankruptcy over medical expenses.

The Honesty Diet

Again, if you choose to value your job or career more than your health, you give up your right to complain about your health. I would ask you to consider, if you choose to value your job more than your health, how are you going to go to work at your job if you are diseased or dead? You may want to reconsider this value of yours. It is literally killing you.

Yeah, but: "Your suggestion is flawed. If everyone moves away from polluted areas, then the less polluted areas will become just as polluted as the area you moved from."

I give you credit for being clever. I even give you credit for *thinking*, but your "Yeah, but" doesn't hold up. It's not honest. You are just pseudo-rationalizing your real objection, which is your desire to not change. Here's why. I am not suggesting *everyone* move away from polluted areas. I am suggesting *you* do. Most people will not take my advice (In fact, most people will *never* read this book). Most people do not value their health. But you can! You can be the beneficiary of others' stupidity, laziness, cowardice and dishonesty. You can move to a cleaner area and be healthier! Don't worry. Most won't.

Big Rock 3: Sleep (Darkness and Sunshine)

The third most important physical requirement for being a healthy human, *still* isn't food… it's sleep. Humans can only go about 12 days at the very most without sleep. Therefore, sleep is the next most important requirement for good health. The primary purpose of sleep isn't just to not be tired, as most people think. It's healing, specifically tissue repair. The majority of our body's regeneration of tissue occurs while we are asleep and when our brain waves are in a particular state, which is induced only after a requisite number of uninterrupted hours of sleep. Because of poor sleeping habits, many people never reach these brain wave states that repair tissue. As such, there is very little healing of body tissue and a much greater chance of obesity, disease, and cancer.

Studies have documented that people who sleep inadequately have a higher incidence of cancer and obesity than those who get high quality sleep. No sleep or poor sleep means early death, fat, and an increased likelihood of disease – something you now know as, fat-sick. Americans are notorious for chronic sleep deprivation and not coincidentally, Americans have terrible health. Other studies have shown that under certain conditions some immunity factors don't even activate until after nine consecutive hours of sleep! How many of us get that much sleep each night? Many Americans, particularly people over fifty-five, get less than six hours per night. This is a primary cause of premature aging, pain, cancer, weight gain, and overall poor health. Therefore, if you really want to improve your health, sleep should take a higher priority than food.

Directly related to sleep are the important notions of darkness and sunshine. People don't usually think of darkness as something related to good health; however, it is critical. In short, inadequate darkness during sleep lessens the repair of tissue and causes the insufficient production and regulation of hormones including melatonin, which, in turn, wreaks havoc on the endocrine system and sets up a cascade of premature aging, weight gain, and overall physiologic collapse.

I sleep in absolute darkness, which is required by the body to produce proper levels of hormones. I take special care to black out all windows and even cover all LED lights emitting from things such as smoke detectors, alarm clocks, televisions, mobile phones and alike.

How long could someone go without darkness? I have no idea, but I do know keeping people in bright light 24 hours a day, day after day, is used as a form of interrogation because of how it messes with physiology and psychology.

The flipside to darkness, of course, is sunshine. The polarity of this relationship is required for the proper function of circadian rhythms, which regulate and modulate innumerable physiologic processes, but primarily those of the endocrine or hormone system. How long could one go without sunshine? In theory, probably years. Of course, we do know chronic darkness causes depression, so maybe not as long as we might think. It is also well documented that, at the time of this writing, most of the American population is already severely vitamin D deficient, a direct result of inadequate exposure to sunshine. Inadequate sunshine is strongly linked to conditions like osteoporosis, depression, heart disease, obesity, high blood pressure and chronic pain. And, as previously mentioned from former Surgeons General, up to 70% of all cancers could be avoided with adequate Vitamin D levels. So sunshine is another important health factor.

However, most conventional health professionals and so-called "health" marketers have successfully convinced the majority of the American population that sunshine is evil. In my opinion, nothing could be further from the truth. While many health professionals espouse the importance of using sun block and avoiding sunshine at all costs, other researchers are documenting the near epidemic of vitamin D deficiency among many Americans. Chronic pain, for example, is at epidemic proportions in the United States. Yet, studies have shown sun exposure stimulates serotonin, has anti-bacterial, anti-viral, and anti-fungal properties, and decreases pain.

Big Rock 4: Food

Finally, only after we have taken *seriously* the first three big rocks of health: air, water, and sleep, do we now get to food! Humans can only go a month or two at the most without food. Isn't it interesting though that when most people try to improve their health, they almost always start with food. Why do people do this? Because it is the easiest area to address and the least invasive to our lifestyle. Addressing the first three big rocks (air, water and sleep) requires more attention, commitment, and discipline; and, of course, Americans always like to do the seemingly easiest things first, like putting things in our mouths because we are so very good at swallowing

The Honesty Diet

things (except the truth). I'm not suggesting that food isn't important. It is one of the big rocks! However, in the hierarchy of physical human needs, air, water, and sleep precede food in importance and should first be addressed for good health.

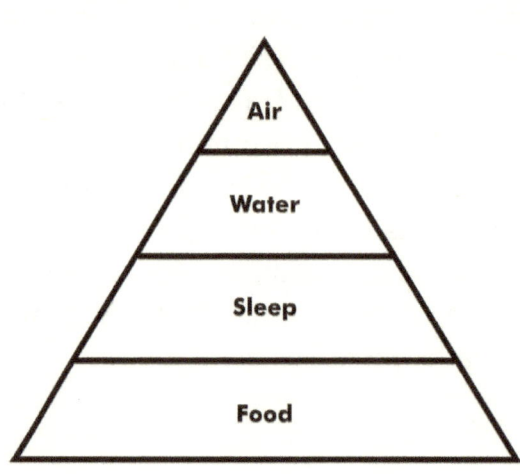

Of course, there are many other important factors for being a healthy human. However, in my opinion, these are the "big rocks" of health. Yet, I contend most Americans ignore at least three, and in many cases, all four of these big rocks of physical health. Many Americans spend their health efforts taking supplements, purchasing exercise equipment advertised on infommericals, wearing "yoga pants" but not actually doing yoga, eating "energy" bars (formerly called "candy bars") and drinking meal replacement shakes – even though none of these are the big rocks of health! These are all dishonest ways of trying to improve your physical health. It is no wonder 66% of Americans are fat! It is no wonder the wealthiest country in the world with the most advanced medical technologies and with the greatest number of doctors is one of the least healthy countries in the world. I have contended throughout this book that this is because we are simultaneously the least *honest* country in the world, as far as it relates to health.

Sources of Energy

We usually think of "energy" in terms of "degree of tiredness," an ability to "get things done" or to be productive. However, it must be recognized that "energy" is actually how we heal and stay healthy. Biochemically, energy is called adenosine triphosphate molecules or "ATP," for short. It is produced in the mitochondria of every cell of the body. Having no ATP means having no energy. No energy means obesity. No energy means having pain. No energy means developing disease. No energy means no healing. Got it?

Earlier I mentioned that while food was a major source of energy, there are other sources of energy. We have just explored those other sources: air, water, and sleep. These come first. Then food. Let's *think* about it. You could say, figuratively, the *hierarchy of physical human needs* is also the *hierarchy of energy* and could be read as:

1. People who can't breathe have no energy. (AIR)
2. People who aren't hydrated have no energy. (WATER)
3. People who don't rest well have no energy. (SLEEP)
4. People who don't eat well have no energy. (FOOD)

The Honesty Diet

Now that we understand this hierarchy of health, let's take a deep dive into the 4th big rock: food, and what people associate most often with the traditional notion of a "diet." Let's also remember to explore food from our newfound perspective of The Honesty Point.

~ 23 ~

FOOD PRINCIPLES OF THE HONESTY DIET

A major problem with nearly all diets is they practically require you to get a degree in nutrition in order to follow them. They frequently require some understanding of biochemistry so you can effectively read labels, avoid harmful ingredients, and calculate complicated formulas and ratios in your head, such as net carbohydrates, calories, and percentage of "good" and "bad" fats. These diets are difficult to follow because they can require cumbersome, mathematical calculation before each and every meal. With The Honesty Diet, you'll probably be happy to hear no such calculations are required.

As we approach the final chapters of this book, you may again be asking yourself, "When is he going to get to the actual diet?" Well, as I've said before, this is the actual diet. If I just told you what specific foods to eat or not eat, then you wouldn't be *thinking* and, therefore, you will have missed the very point and very essence of this book. Everyone lives life at a different level of honesty and, therefore, the diet is different for everyone. The diet is unique to each individual and is based on each individual's own level of honesty at any given point in time. Instead, I am going to share with you several principles I hold for myself – at least at the time of this writing. I offer such principles only as an example to help you forge your own. No doubt, as my understanding of the Honesty Diet deepens, I, too, will adjust my own principles accordingly.

The Honesty Diet is a personal, dynamic, ever-refining process. The number of principles you will hold for yourself most likely change over time in direct proportion to the degree to which you are being honest with yourself. Some of your principles may seem honest at one point in your life, but as your level of honesty, awareness, and visceral intelligence increases, they may be eliminated, changed, or evolve at a later point in your life.

If you aren't getting the results you seek, then you only need to reexamine your principles and become more honest with yourself. Don't be afraid to ask for help from others. Friends, family, and *thinking* health professionals can be excellent resources for helping you see yourself in a more honest light. These principles only require a willingness to exhibit honesty while shopping for food, selecting a meal at a restaurant, or preparing a meal at home. You are more than welcome to add to, subtract from, or alter all of the following – except the first principle. To get any meaningful results, Principle One is required.

Principle 1: Be Honest and Think!

I have already devoted much of this book to this first principle, because it is the principle upon which The Honesty Diet rests. Without this first principle, others won't have much value. Although Principle One is a simple principle, it isn't necessarily an easy principle for most to accept. In fact, because of America's socially-conditioned medical captivity, Principle One may be the most challenging principle to actually put into practice. Remember: I contend the primary cause of obesity, poor health, chronic pain, and most disease in the United States is *dishonesty*. If you want to improve your health, it will require transcending to a higher level of self-honesty. Recognize and accept the fact that your current level of health is a product of, and is directly proportional to, your current level of honesty.

Principle 2: Eat More Water, Don't Drink More Water!

We introduced this principle earlier. However, now would be a good time to expand the concept. Water foods, again, are almost exclusively fruits and vegetables – preferably organic fruits and vegetables.

Many health professionals spout off the old wives' tale, "everyone should drink eight, 8-ounce glasses of water each day." The only problem is there isn't really any evidence to support this assertion. That much water may even harm your kidneys. The origin of this old wives' tale appears to be the misinterpretation of a government study from the 1950s. That study concluded the average person

The Honesty Diet

should consume the *equivalent* of eight, 8-ounce glasses of water per day. But, the study went on to emphasize that the *overwhelming majority* of water should come from eating food, *not from drinking water*!

I know people who spend half their day trying to keep track of how many glasses of water they drink, or they carry a giant 64-ounce plastic container around with them and spend the other half of their day in the bathroom urinating. Let's *think* for a minute. If you are drinking water all day long and spending a good part of your day urinating, does that really sound like you are *hydrating* yourself? If you drink 64 ounces and urinate 60 ounces, is that hydration? I don't think so. It sounds to me like you are just passing water through your body with very little absorption. If you were actually hydrating yourself, I would think you wouldn't have to pee all day. Doesn't that make sense?

If you are not used to eating water, it can be a somewhat unpleasant experience to just rush out and start eating lots of fruits and vegetables all at once. Your body may initially rebel because, in general, the body doesn't like sudden change or anything it isn't already accustomed to.

I suggested eating more water to one person who immediately attempted to eat the way I was eating. He later complained he spent the entire day on the toilet with diarrhea. Of course, he did! He tried to change his hydration level overnight and his body objected. So be sure to gradually build up your consumption of water-foods.

Yeah, but: "I hate fruits and vegetables."

Now, if you say you hate the taste of fruits and vegetables – that is a symptom. Hating the taste of fruits and vegetables is the number one, telltale sign of a sugar addict – a junkie, if you will. If you hate the taste of fruits and vegetables, you have a serious addiction that needs to be broken immediately. If you don't *want* to break your addiction to sugar – if you don't have any desire to break the addiction – that's even stronger evidence of your junkie status.

Sometimes a person is so addicted to something they can't even recognize their addiction. There is an old saying – "Fish discover water last," which means even though fish spend their entire lives in water, they may be unaware of water's existence because they have no other experience other than being in water. Only when a fish is pulled out of the water by a fisherman's hook or net does a fish finally realize water exists! Sugar addicts are very much like a fish in water. They are so addicted to sugar, they can't recognize their addiction.

In addition to hating the taste of fruits and vegetables, sugar addicts have a tendency to say things like, "I don't like the taste of water." These people are in serious, serious trouble. The more sugar a person consumes, especially in unnatural forms such as high fructose corn syrup and artificial sweeteners, the more they tend to dislike the taste of water and *real* foods like fruits and vegetables. Healthy-thinking people *want* to break their adverse addictions. Unhealthy-thinking people *rarely* want to break their addictions. Their poor health is a self-evident, self-fulfilling prophecy.

The Honesty Diet

Your body was evolutionarily designed to consume fruits and vegetables. Fruits and vegetables are a primary source of energy for the human physiology. They are the ideal fuels for your engine (although, I don't necessarily advocate vegetarianism). If you try to run your unleaded car engine (your body) on diesel fuel (fast-food, junk food, etc.), it may run for a while, but it is going to sputter, break down, and die much sooner than it is supposed to. It will also be a painful process.

Yeah, but: "I don't need to eat fruits and vegetables. I just listen to my body."

Many people say things like, "I just trust and listen to my body. If something doesn't sound or taste good to me, then I don't eat it." What they mean is, if their body doesn't like something, it must not be good for them. This is their attempted means of eating "naturally" and claiming to listen to their body's internal wisdom. Normally, this is an acceptable philosophy toward selecting foods. However, it only works if a person does not have any adverse addictions to something they consume.

Most people, as we have already thoroughly discussed, have many adverse food addictions skewing their body's sense of what does and does not taste good. Before one can trust any cravings or aversions to various foods like fruits and vegetables, one must first break addictions to the things severely skewing one's sense of taste, such as excessive sugar, coffee, cigarettes, soft drinks, fast-food and other processed foods. Many of these same individuals would also contend if something made them feel bloated, they wouldn't eat it; since their body was rejecting it, it probably wasn't good for them. However, this is unlikely to be the case. It is much more likely the body would initially reject something like fruits and vegetables because the body had become accustomed to being dehydrated, even though dehydration is *causing* or will cause some of their health problems.

Yeah, but: "Doesn't eating fruits and vegetables taste terrible?"

No. Like anything else, after a while, your body accepts the food as normal and then actually begins to *create* specific cravings for fruits and vegetables. This is a function and process of addiction like any other. How do you think you came to love waffles, pancakes and home fries for breakfast? – Simply by developing an *addiction* to it. I know to some this assertion sounds unlikely, but it is true. It only sounds absurd because of your addiction. If you are an addict, you can't see how this is true. You can only learn it and understand it through experience. You can *choose* to develop the same addiction to water foods like fruits and vegetables, if you really *want* to. It isn't hard, either. In fact, once your body gets a taste of being hydrated, it will *crave* water foods throughout the day and it will crave less food overall.

Yeah, but: "Organic produce is too expensive. I don't have the money for that."

Again, something is only expensive if you don't *value* it. If organic produce seems too expensive, that is usually a good indication you don't *value* organic produce. You don't value it because you have a lower awareness of how organic produce can benefit your health. You don't value it because organic produce doesn't have *more meaning* to you than conventional produce. However, I recommend you just try it for a month or two. Then you can decide if it's still too expensive. Furthermore, the idea organic produce is too expensive is a common misconception. In my experience, organic foods cost less than conventional foods. I'll explain why shortly.

Yeah, but: "I don't need to eat fruits and vegetables. I get my daily nutrients from supplements."

A fellow doctor I once met boasted to me that he eats *at least* 15 servings of fruits and vegetables per day. Wow! I thought. That's more than I usually eat. He must be really healthy! Oddly, though, he didn't look healthy. He then proceeded to tell me he actually takes daily supplements made of dehydrated fruits and vegetables. Oh, I thought. That's not very honest. That's not *really* eating 15 servings of fruits and vegetables per day. These supplements have been pressed into a powder and encapsulated into pill form. He claims they are the *equivalent* of 15 servings of fruits and vegetables. Of course, he then suggested I should take them, too, and tried to sell them to me. I declined.

This doctor was lying. He wasn't being honest with himself. He said to me, "I eat 15 servings per day *and that's on top of whatever else I eat!*" Clearly, he was very proud of his consumptive statistic. However, I'd be willing to bet this doctor almost never eats an actual fruit or vegetable. He just lies to himself and tells himself that he eats 15 servings per day just because he pops a few supplements each morning. This is dishonest. A *thinking* doctor would know that much of the benefit is found in the water and fiber content of any given fruit or vegetable. Even more benefit is found in the *synergy* between the water content, the fiber content, and the vitamins, minerals, and other micronutrients contained within. Swallowing dehydrated fruits and vegetables removes *almost all* of the benefit, in my opinion. We must remember these products are called *supplements*, not *substitutes*! Yet, that is exactly how this doctor and many other people treat such supplements, as *substitutes* for real food! This doesn't work.

Supplements aren't bad. I take many. However, I don't lie about it. I don't kid myself into thinking that taking supplements means I don't have to eat properly. Most people abuse supplements. They take supplements and think they don't have to eat healthy foods like fruits and vegetables. That's cheating, and it's dishonest. Interestingly enough, most people who've tried to sell me supplements aren't very fit or healthy looking. In fact, many of them are flat out fat-sick. I wonder why that is? Maybe it's because those attracted to such a method for achieving health are fundamentally lazy people always looking to cut corners.

Principle 3: Don't Confuse "Full" With "Nourished"

I am convinced one of the reasons Americans overeat so much is because they confuse the sensation of being "full" with being "nourished." Understanding the difference between these two sensations is not something easily explained or described. You can't learn this distinction *intellectually*. You must experience it *viscerally*. It is like trying to describe chocolate to someone who has never had chocolate before. You can't explain it. It must be experienced. However, once experienced, your visceral intelligence increases exponentially.

How does the body let us know it needs nourishment? It produces sensations of *hunger*. The body is a lot like a crying baby. An infant can't easily communicate that it's hungry, in pain, or needs to be changed. A baby only does one thing: it cries. Similarly, the body can't tell you *exactly* what food it needs. It, too, does only one thing: it cries through hunger pangs. That is how the body informs you that you're hungry. Sure, you could argue that the body, to some extent, can communicate specific cravings, but even that "language" isn't terribly specific.

When people feel hungry, most think it's because their stomach is *empty* and, therefore, needs to be *filled*. This is dead wrong. Hunger doesn't mean your stomach needs to be *filled*. Hunger means your body needs *nourishment*. Nourishment means eating *real* food. When you choose to eat *fake* foods, like meal replacement shakes, energy bars (again, I mean candy bars), fast-food or junk food, you may be *eating*, but you're not necessarily eating *real* food. You're just putting things in your body that may look like food and may even smell and taste like what you've come to call food, but it certainly isn't *real* food. Rarely do people choose to eat foods providing them with *nourishment* – what their hunger sensations are screaming for in the first place.

Normal Hunger Progression

Hunger ➔ "Real" Food ➔ Nourished Sensation ➔ Satisfied

When most people feel hungry, instead of eating real food, i.e. something natural and nutritious, most people grab some junky, highly processed fat food. Oops! I mean, "fast" food (Sorry, Freudian slip, I suppose). They'll *fill* their stomachs to more than 100% of normal capacity, thinking that will satisfy their hunger. Then, less than an hour or two later, they often feel hungry again, so they repeat the process by snacking on some more highly-processed, trans-fat-rich snacks. But, honestly, do you think their bodies have gotten what they sought? Has the body gotten what it needed? Was the reason they felt hungry so soon after eating because there weren't enough French fries or energy bars in their stomachs? No. Within an hour or two the body again tries to convey it still needs nourishment, creates the same hunger sensations, and the person, in turn, eats the wrong stuff again. The stomach didn't need to be *filled*. The body needed to be *nourished* with real food.

The Honesty Diet

As stated before, these are not the same things. Like an infant who can only communicate by crying, the body continues to "cry" through hunger sensations, begging for *nourishment* until it gets some. As a result, a person just keeps on eating, becoming fatter and fatter.

For many, this vicious cycle continues endlessly throughout the day. Then people have the audacity to wonder why they're so fat.

Hunger's Vicious Cycle

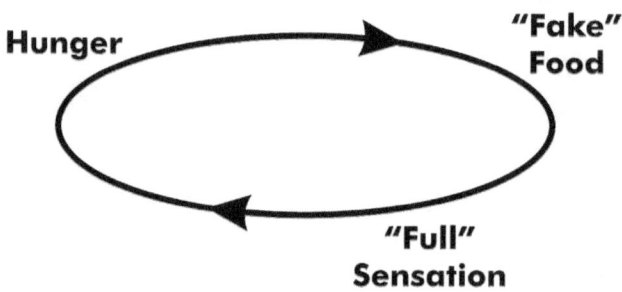

You continue to be hungry all the time because you're feeding your body the wrong things. You're "filling" your stomach with *fake* foods that don't provide the nourishment the body requires. People stuck in this cycle aren't being honest with themselves. They aren't paying attention to their body's needs and messages. So, what should you eat? What does your body really need? What is nourishment? You already know the answers to these questions if you are being *honest* with yourself.

Stress and Fat

If *nourishment* were withheld from you for extended periods of time, would that stress you out a bit? Would that stress you out a lot? Of course, it would. When the body is stressed, it produces that previously discussed sympathetic neurological state known as "fight or flight." When the body is in this stressed-out state it reverts to its most basic, primary function of survival. If the body thinks it must go into survival mode because of chronic stress it will store any form of calories – as fat. The body very intelligently does this in the event it is unable to find *nourishment* in the future.

Americans are almost never at a loss for finding things to eat, but they are *starving* for nourishment – hence the chronic weight gain. This chronic weight-gaining phenomenon is a basic survival mechanism. Since fat food (again, I mean "fast"-food) is not *real* food, the body is robbed of *nourishment*. This produces a state of stress, which *causes* fat storage. This is why many people can't lose weight. They don't eat *real* food! People must recognize hunger as a signal that the body needs *nourishment* – not that the stomach needs to be *filled*. Fast-food, junk food, and fake food are not nourishment. Giving the stomach a feeling of "fullness" does not satisfy the body's hunger. If you want to nourish your body and lose weight, you have to eat *real* food. Therefore, the new awareness is:

*The more fake food you eat,
the fatter you become.*

If something is a *real* food then it provides nourishment. If something does not provide nourishment, then it is not a food. Therefore, fast-food French fries are not food because they don't provide nourishment. If you were to use a "Yeah, but" and suggest French fries are potatoes and, therefore, provide *some* nourishment, you'd be using French fries as a language lie, and you would be being dishonest with yourself. French fries, under most circumstances, contain massive amounts of trans-fats and other non-food additives. They are not food. For a number of reasons, they make you fat.

How Much Should You Eat?

Not feeling "full" doesn't mean you feel "hungry" all the time. There is a big space between full and empty. It's kind of like a tank of gas for your car. Most of the time, you are neither full, nor empty. Most of the time, you are somewhere in between. Like a gas tank, that's how you want your stomach to be, too – a quarter-tank full, a half-tank full, three-quarters full, etc. The goal should never be to "Fill 'er up!" A car works just as well with a half tank of gas as it does with a full tank of gas. Just remember:

> *Every time you feel "full"*
> *you're getting fatter.*

Portion Control Is Not the Answer

There is a lot of talk today about portion control. The perception exists that if we would just eat smaller portions we could lose weight and be healthier. I disagree. Portion control is a red herring. Portion size isn't the real problem. In order to understand why portion size is excessive in the United States, we must *think* and ask *why* are people eating such large portions at meals? The reason is because what they are being served isn't food! The more stuff you choose to eat that isn't food, the larger your portion sizes will tend to be. Why? Because when you choose to eat fake food, when you haven't fed the body nourishment – you haven't fed it real food, your body continues to say it's hungry. Remember: don't confuse being full with being nourished.

Forcing portion control on society does not work, will not work, and it cannot work for most people because it *doesn't address hunger*. Trying to eat smaller portions of fake food at meals doesn't do anything about the hunger. *Starvation* is the reason so many people in the United States eat so much. Within reason, you don't really have to worry about portion control if you'll just choose to eat real foods instead of fake foods. The recently popular contention of portion control as a means of losing weight is wasted effort in most cases. Having said that, please also remember men tend to be bigger than women and have different metabolisms. So ladies, I encourage you to remember and repeat this epigram:

If you eat as much as your man,
you're going to weigh as much as your man!

Principle 4: Eat Food, Not Doof™

In Principle Three, I made reference to real foods and fake foods. So, now we need to define specifically what each are. I contend everybody already knows the difference between real foods and fake food... if they are practicing Principle One. However, I understand that for most people their addiction to and disease of medical captivity is so severe they have literally forgotten how to tell a real food from a fake food.

I hesitate to refer to things like fast-food, soft drinks, coffee, energy bars, and other edibles as "food" for one simple reason: *They aren't food*! Today, many of us are afraid to eat some of the most nutritious foods such as eggs and avocados. Yet, we consistently choose to eat the least nutritious foods like fast-food chicken, pizza, burgers, French fries, and tacos from famous fat food chains.

In many ways, people in the United States have it completely backwards and insist upon eating the very opposite of food on a daily basis. I never really knew what to call it – eating the very *opposite* of food – so I simply termed it *"doof,"* which is "food" spelled backward. Most Americans eat doof, not food, all day long. They then have the audacity to wonder why they are so fat-sick!

People often ask me what foods to eat. "Should I eat meat?" "Should I eat eggs?" "Should I avoid carbohydrates?" "Should I avoid fats?" "Should I drink protein shakes?" My answer was always the same: Be honest, *think*, and eat *food*. Our medical captivity has robbed most of us of our ability to think for ourselves and determine what is and what is not *real* food. The irony is that distinguishing between what is *food* and what is *doof* escapes us, not because it's complicated, but because we are just out of practice of doing so. Principle Four teaches us a simple methodology providing a greater insight into the current level of honesty and awareness we have about our food choices.

Let's practice Principle One for a moment. Be honest and *think*. Your body is designed to run on what? *Food*. Your body takes in *food*, breaks it down, burns it for energy and rebuilds your body with it. That is basically how your body's food intake system works. If you eat things other than *food* – that is, if you eat *doof* – your body can't break it down and burn it as energy… at least not very well! Therefore, one of the major reasons people become fat-sick is because they don't eat *food*. Your body is not designed to run on artificial chemicals and highly-processed *doof*. So, don't eat that stuff! *It isn't food*! Again, you don't put diesel fuel in a car that runs on unleaded gasoline. If you do, you will quickly wreck the engine. Have the same respect for your body. Otherwise, you'll wreck that quickly, too.

It is not a coincidence that in the United States Type II diabetes has reached epidemic levels in direct correlation with the introduction of doof to the American food supply. The onset of Type II diabetes and many other degenerative diseases is a strong indication of a wrecked digestive system – an abused digestive system, a doof-laden digestive system. So, eat *real* food.

The Honesty Diet

> *"Americans... are fatally attracted to the slow death of fast-food."*
>
> – Comedian, George Carlin

The *food/doof* methodology can apply not only to finished, ready-to-eat foods, but to specific ingredients as well. For example, most people don't usually think of salt as a food, but, of course, it is a common food substance or food ingredient. Put on your honesty glasses again for a minute and try the following exercise. Identify each of the following as either *food* or *doof*. Believe it or not, it may be harder than you think.

1. Fruits
2. Vegetables
3. Eggs
4. Avocados
5. Sugar
6. Salt
7. Fat
8. French fries
9. Salt substitute
10. Sugar substitute
11. Protein powder
12. High fructose corn syrup
13. Trans-fat

Don't Take Advice From Fat Doctors!

In the above exercise, items 1-7 are food. Items 8-13 are doof. This shouldn't be a difficult exercise, but is for some. You'd be surprised at how many people label things like sugar, salt, avocados and fat as unhealthy doof! They're not. These are real, natural, and dare I say, "healthy" foods. *Think* about it. Fat is natural. Trans-fat is fake. Sugar is natural. Sugar substitute is fake. Salt is natural. Salt substitute is fake. Fake foods are not foods. They are *doof* and, again, your body is not designed to break down and burn fake foods. *Don't eat them!*

I actually know people who would never touch an egg because, according to them, it contains *evil* cholesterol, but then they will regularly eat greasy fast-food and other doof-like energy bars, and they'll use artificial salt and artificial sugar. *How stupid is this?* We have been so brainwashed by companies marketing so-called "health" foods, and by doctors with little or no nutritional education that we actually are afraid of *real* foods like fat, sugar, salt, eggs, and avocados. Many of us actually believe nonfat foods, sugar substitutes, and salt substitutes are healthier for us than real foods. How incredibly sad.

To help get you back into the habit of *thinking*, do the following exercise: for the next seven days, before putting *anything edible* in your mouth, ask yourself whether what you are eating is food or doof. Believe it or not, just raising your awareness to this basic level of honesty can dramatically improve your diet, your health, and help you lose weight. This, again, is a function of the Observer Effect discussed in an early chapter: *the mere observation of an event changes the event itself.* Don't complicate things. Acknowledge you are not fat because you eat too much food. Acknowledge you are fat because you eat too much *doof*! Honestly, you shouldn't eat *any* doof, but I trust you get the point.

No System Is Bulletproof

Now, obviously this system or technique for identifying something as food or doof isn't bulletproof. For example, fruit juice could be considered food if it is 100% juice, or it could also be considered doof if it were only 8% juice and 92% high fructose corn syrup and water. *Whether or not this is considered food or doof depends largely on your degree of inward honesty.* What if an item contains 98% food ingredients and only 2% doof ingredients? Is it food or doof? The answer, again, would depend upon your health goals, your values, and your degree of inward honesty. It's up to you. I suggest you go look in the mirror again, evaluate your body, and then make your decision accordingly. Some people might choose to eat a food item and justify it by saying, "It's only 2% doof." However, what if a food item was only 2% arsenic, 2% mercury or 2% lead? Would you still eat it? Well, for my own health, I recognize doof is just as dangerous and harmful to my health and fitness as arsenic, mercury, or lead.

Here is a technique I use to help me determine whether or not something is food or doof. Remember the childhood game Rock, Paper, Scissors? Two people each shake a closed fist, count to three, then show to the other person a hand symbol for "rock" – a closed fist, "paper" – an open hand, or "scissors" – two spread-open fingers. The rules are: scissors cut paper; rock smashes scissors; and *paper covers rock*. It is just a silly game, but I have found it handy for helping me determine whether or not I should eat something. I pretend the food item is the "rock," and "paper" is doof. In the game's rules paper covers rock. Or, in this case, *doof covers food*. That means, I have decided that, in general, any food item containing doof or doof ingredients is simply doof – *no matter how much or how little doof is in the item*. If a "food" item is 95% food and only 5% doof, it doesn't matter – *paper covers rock* – it is deemed doof. Therefore, I don't eat it.

For example, French fries may be made mostly of potatoes, which, of course, are food. However, since the French fries of most fat-food restaurants are made with partially-hydrogenated oils (a.k.a. trans-fats) that cause obesity and disease, I never eat them. See? Paper covers rock – doof covers food. I recognize and understand that doof is so dangerous to my health I make every effort to refrain from eating any items I know contain any amount of doof. Most people don't understand this. And, that is largely why they are so fat-sick. They eat doof!

Principle 5: Your Refrigerator Is Your Body

Let me show you how to see inside your body without any hi-tech medical equipment. Go to your refrigerator right now. Open the door, look inside, and tell me what you see. Whatever you see inside your refrigerator and your pantry is what your body is made out of. If you see food like organic fruits and vegetables, and organic meats and cheeses, then that is what your body is made out of. If you see soda, beer, fast-food leftovers, potato chips and ice cream, then *that* is exactly what your body is made out of. Is your body made of organic, healthy food? Or is your body made of greasy fast-food, junk food, and other doof? Which of these two bodies is less likely to be fat? Which is less likely to be sick? Which is less likely to grow cancer? Which is less likely to be in pain? If you are practicing the Honesty Diet, you already know the answers to these questions.

The new awareness, then, is:

Your Refrigerator = Your Body

Now ask yourself this question: What are your children made of? Again, whatever is in your refrigerator and your pantry is what your children's bodies are made of. Are your children made of doof or food? Are your children made of soda? Candy? Chocolate? Cookies? If so, are you *really* being a good parent? Are your children really going to grow up to be strong, healthy, fit, intelligent, attractive, emotionally-competent adults with what is currently in your refrigerator and pantry? If your children won't eat anything else but the doof in your pantry, is it because they really don't like healthy food? Or, have you just let them become young, addicted junkies? Be honest. What is the truth about the situation?

Your Refrigerator = Your Children's Bodies

Don't Take Advice From Fat Doctors!

Principle 6: Eat Those *In*expensive Organic Foods

Many health experts assert that buying organic food is cheaper *in the long run*. When I speak to people about buying organic foods, the most common "Yeah, but" I hear is they can't buy organic foods because organic foods are too expensive. "Do you know what is really expensive? – radiation and chemotherapy!" I only somewhat jest. While some may think this is not a fair comparison, I disagree. Eating organic foods significantly decreases your risk of developing many different kinds of common cancers. And, while this may not yet be demonstrable with long-term, double-blind, placebo-controlled, randomized human clinical trials involving tens of thousands of people (as most studies on any subject do not), there is some promising animal and experimental research suggesting this assertion is, in fact, true. More importantly, the presence or absence of such research is irrelevant. *Thinking* is sufficient enough to prove this assertion.

I certainly agree with the notion that buying organic food is cheaper in the long run. However, it is my experience buying organic foods is also cheaper *in the short run*! A few years ago, I decided to make every effort to only buy certified organic foods. At first I was concerned that maybe I shouldn't. In some stores, it seemed organic foods were, on average, 50 to 100% more expensive than conventionally-grown foods.

Within a few months, I experienced a really big surprise – a huge savings! My total monthly food bill had actually *decreased* on average by more than 30% since going organic! I had been spending about $1,000 per month on food. Food included groceries and dining out expenses. After about one year of buying organic foods almost exclusively, my total food bill plummeted to around $700 per month. A $300 per month savings! That's a total savings of $3,600 per year!

How did this happen? I began to focus on organic, water-rich foods like fruits and vegetables. I was literally eating eight to ten or more servings of water-rich fruits and vegetables per day, every day! This habit substantially increased the amount of fiber in my diet. It also hydrated my body more than I ever thought possible. I subsequently realized that – without trying – I was eating much less food, overall. I contend it was because the organic foods I was consuming contained many more nutrients than conventional foods, and fewer contaminants like pesticides, fungicides, hormones, and antibiotics. As a result, I was less hungry because my body was *nourished*. I now eat much less food than I used to, and my grocery bill has plummeted as a result. I didn't think I was overeating, but clearly I was.

It should be noted I don't punish myself, and I do not suffer by not enjoying food. Quite to the contrary, I have successfully reprogrammed my body back to where it's supposed to be, craving healthy, nourishing foods instead of grease-laden, trans-fat foods that so many fat-sick Americans crave and can't go more than a single day without. Interestingly enough, shortly after making this discovery, I came across an interesting quote in a holistic nutrition text book that helped explain my grocery experience.

Don't Take Advice From Fat Doctors!

> *"Live foods have so much nourishment in them that considerably less food is needed to get the same amount of nutrition... As we become healthy, we often require less food because the body is better able to assimilate the physical aspects of the food and the more subtle energies from which the food is condensed."*
>
> – Author, Dr. Gabriel Cousins

As a result of going almost completely organic, I feel more energetic, I lost weight without trying (not that I necessarily needed to by most people's standards, but obviously I did have weight to lose), I eat better, spend less, and I no longer crave going out to dinner several times per week. I still go out to restaurants, but it's more a social activity with family or friends than it is an eating activity. This is clear evidence, albeit anecdotal, demolishing the assertion that organic food is "too expensive." My new awareness, quite to my delight and surprise, is buying organic foods has put an additional $300 per month in my pocket! If a dollar saved is a dollar earned, then for me, buying organic foods makes me money, it doesn't cost me money! Truly I have demonstrated and experienced that buying organic is better for me in the long run and in the short run!

One of the fastest ways to lose weight healthfully is to eat more organic foods. Organic foods nourish your body. When your body is *nourished* it isn't hungry all the time. You eat less food overall and you lose weight naturally, healthfully, and without really trying. All you have to do is decide and then start to purchase more organic foods. Doing so is cheaper than buying nutritionless conventional foods.

By the way, did you notice the language lie I glazed over in the above paragraph? We all may understand what "organic" produce is. But, what about that other term we use nowadays? What in the world is "conventional" produce or "conventionally-grown" produce? Technically, "conventional" means the produce may have been grown or transported with chemical pesticides and herbicides or it may be genetically modified in some way.

In other words – in more honest words – it means the produce may be *toxic*. But we don't label the food as toxic, do we? You've never seen a sign in the grocery store aisle reading the "Toxic Produce" section. No. Instead, we soften the truth with language lies so we don't feel bad about what we are purchasing and putting into our bodies, and we call those sections "conventional" or "conventionally-grown""produce sections. Just remember, conventional produce often means toxic produce. The term "conventional" is simply a language lie.

Principle 7: Read Labels Carefully

"Organic" Isn't Always "Healthy"

Now I know we just spent a considerable amount of time discussing the value of organic foods. However, organic doesn't always mean healthy. In the past decade or so, the term "organic" has become a household term. Some

Don't Take Advice From Fat Doctors!

major supermarkets have even introduced their own brand of organic foods. I commend them for this effort. However, just because something is labeled organic doesn't necessarily mean it is a real food. Something organic can still be doof, albeit "organic" doof.

The term "organic" is not a free pass for eating just anything. In the past year, I have come across a number of "organic" products that are still doof. Organic chocolate cookies with vanilla frosting cream center, for example, are still doof even if they are made with organic ingredients. Be honest. *Are cookies food*? No. Then don't eat them. Don't lie to yourself that just because they're made from organic ingredients they *must* be healthy. They're not. There're still cookies!

Consumers, in their attempts to eat healthier, are still going to be conned if they're not careful and honest. I even became a victim of this marketing manipulation not too long ago. I was thrilled when I came across an organic mixed berry juice. I quickly purchased the item and took it home. Upon first tasting it, I realized my error. It tasted terribly sweet – artificially sweet. I looked more carefully at the label and saw the words "contains 10% juice." *Damn*, I thought. *They got me*. I had just bought doof – organic doof.

Reading the ingredients, I found the manufacturers weren't technically lying. All of the ingredients were "organic." However, the juice cocktail was full of "organic cane sugar" which isn't much different from the nonorganic garbage juices available in the same aisle of the store. Maybe you could argue this product is a little healthier, but not much – certainly not enough to qualify as *doof*-less. I know earlier we talked about how sugar is a real food and shouldn't be feared. However, excessive sugar, even if it is organic sugar, isn't healthy. Of course, a sugar substitute would have been even less healthy.

Just be careful and be honest. Just because it's labeled organic, doesn't necessarily make it healthy. Read the labels.

"Natural" Can Be a Dangerous Term

The word "natural" has become a legal language lie marketers use to try to make their product appear healthy to eat. Today, it seems every edible item for sale has the word "natural" printed on the packaging. Through the passing of various laws pertaining to food labeling, the word "natural" has come to mean, in essence, anything that comes from planet Earth is technically natural. Therefore, natural has become a fairly meaningless term in the health food industry.

In my experience, when a company prominently advertises their product is made from "all natural ingredients," that is usually a good sign I probably *shouldn't* eat the item. For example, which is an *honest* use of the term "natural" – natural chicken or natural soda? Obviously, if you were practicing honesty, natural chicken would be a more proper use of the word natural. That is not to say "natural" chicken is necessarily healthy for you. It, too, could still contain additives like arsenic (which is natural), as well as other processing, which would make it doof. However, soda, no matter how you think about it, isn't natural and is *always* doof. Still, this doesn't stop people from buying giant cases of "natural" soda at their local wholesale club, and dishonestly convincing themselves they are making healthier food decisions. They aren't. They're just lying to themselves while they become fatter and sicker.

Here is an example of what I mean by natural being a dangerous term. In the past few years, an acquaintance of mine has been making a concerted effort to purchase more healthy foods. One day while visiting her she offered me some potato chips she had bought at the store. "They're healthy! See? It says on the label they're *All Natural!*" She said this with great enthusiasm. I ate a few. They tasted really good... too good... artificially good. I turned the bag over to read the ingredient label. One of the first ingredients was partially-hydrogenated vegetable oil. That's right. These "All Natural" potato chips were chock full of trans-fats. They were neither natural, nor healthy. In fact, these potato chips were one of the least healthy things (doof) one could possibly eat.

I certainly didn't want to embarrass her. She had done nothing wrong. She had just been duped by a disingenuous marketing ploy, just as I had been duped with the organic mixed berry juice. I then explained to her why, although they may meet the legal definition of "natural" for an edible substance in the United States, that didn't at all mean these were healthy potato chips. I then wrote down for her the name of a brand of delicious organic chips she might enjoy instead.

I wonder how many millions of Americans are eating doof cleverly disguised as "health foods." This can be easily avoided with about an hour's worth of

The Honesty Diet

education. However, it takes a genuine desire to learn the information, and most people don't really want to. Most people are perfectly content to buy unhealthy foods disguised as healthy foods, just so they can lie to themselves and pretend they're being health conscious. Not coincidentally, most people in this country remain fat-sick.

> *"Everything is part of nature – nuclear waste, that's part of nature, too!"*
>
> – Comedian, George Carlin

I agree with George – one of the greatest *thinkers* of all time, by the way. Natural is a useless term because everything is natural. Arsenic, mercury, and lead are natural, too. But they are still toxic to humans. I wouldn't recommend eating them. Try to avoid eating items which generously promote the word "Natural" on the packaging. In general, the bigger the word "Natural" the less likely what's inside is to be healthy.

Principle 8: The Fewer Ingredients the Better

In general, the fewer ingredients an item lists on the label, the more healthy the item is likely to be for you. Similarly, the more ingredients listed, the more doof it is likely to contain, and therefore the worse the item tends to be for you. I try to only buy packaged items having about seven or less ingredients listed on the label. If I pick up something with twenty-some-odd ingredients, many of which I often have difficulty pronouncing, I almost never buy the item. You may want to do the same.

If you have difficulty pronouncing a food item's ingredients, you probably shouldn't eat it!

Yeah, but: "Well, then... what can I eat!?"

When I work with people on how to improve their diet, I often hear this: "Well, it sounds like I can't eat anything anymore." I don't know why people feel this way. I don't eat *doof*, and I *never* have any trouble finding things to eat. I occasionally eat meat, but it's organic meat. I eat fruits, nuts, vegetables, and beans, but they are organic. I eat minimal amounts of cheese and breads, but they are organic also. There's plenty to eat. I have come to realize what this objection really means is: *I'm an addict to doof and I don't want to change. I don't like being fat and sick, but giving up my addiction is more painful than remaining fat and sick.* There is absolutely nothing wrong with a choice like this. In fact, it is honest to recognize your thoughts in this way. However, there is a consequence to that decision. You are going to be fat-sick. Therefore, if you make the decision to indulge your addictions and continue to eat doof, you give up your right to legitimately complain about your obesity, diabetes, heart disease, chronic pain, or cancer later.

The Honesty Diet

Principle 9: Avoid "Everything in Moderation"

The slogan "everything in moderation" is popular among many people. But, have you ever really observed people who use this slogan? Do they ever look like they actually *practice* moderation? In my experience, nearly everyone who uses this phrase has a very indulgent-looking body. People who say "everything in moderation" are almost always fat-sick. Coincidence? I don't think so. "Everything in moderation" is a fat-sick person's slogan used to justify habits and choices people intuitively know they shouldn't engage in.

Let's look at what the moderation slogan really means, shall we? Everything in moderation. Really? Everything? Does it mean you should eat a synthetic, man-made substance, like trans-fat, *in moderation*? Does it mean eat pesticides and steroid hormones known to cause disease, in moderation? Does it mean to smoke cigarettes *in moderation*? Does it mean consume high fructose corn syrup in moderation? How about in reference to states of disease? Is a *moderate* case of heart disease healthy? Should we strive for cancer in moderation? Is a moderate case of ADD/ADHD something to strive for? Is HIV *in moderation* a good thing? How about social conditions? Is pollution *in moderation*, OK? Is hate crime *in moderation*, OK? Is slavery *in moderation* acceptable?

Do you see where I am going with this? This slogan, this philosophy of "everything in moderation," is a destructive one. Where, then, did this "everything in moderation" philosophy come from? The only logical answer is this is a philosophy developed by people who didn't *want* to change their unhealthy habits, and who, on some level, knew they should. "Everything in moderation" is a dishonest philosophy and, therefore, has no place in The Honesty Diet.

We as a society have completely lost touch with the concept of "moderation." There are people out there who think "everything in moderation" means things like drinking only one soft drink per day. That isn't moderate. In my opinion, one every day is extremely excessive! A "moderate" amount of soda consumption ought to be something like no more than one or two per month. Or, depending upon your personal level of honesty and awareness, none at all. If we are being honest, we all know soda consumption is incredibly unhealthy. It is one of the worst possible things you can consume. But I think most unhealthy people would suggest that one soda per day is "moderate" consumption. Others think smoking one pack of cigarettes per week is smoking in moderation, but clearly, that's excessive!

But suddenly when it comes to *healthy* activities, these "everything in moderation" people use the very same logic. "I don't want to exercise every day," they said. "That's excessive! Maybe one or two times per week, but not every day – everything in moderation, right?" Do you see how "everything in moderation" is a garbage excuse fat-sick people use to justify their bad habits and try to pass them off as healthy?

"Everything in moderation" has no place and no value in the Honesty Diet.

Principle 10: Eat a "Healthy," Not "Balanced" Diet

Obviously, a *healthy* diet is your objective. If you are fat, you obviously aren't eating a healthy diet. You'd better face up to it now. The proof is in the pudding – or the fat, in this case. If you are fat, you are eating too much food, too much doof, or both. If you'll just be honest with yourself, then you can get fit and healthy. Stay dishonest and you will stay fat, sick, and in pain.

However, a *healthy* diet should never be confused with America's warped perception and misuse of a *balanced* diet. For decades, doctors told their patients to eat a "balanced" diet. They gave this advice largely because allopathically-trained doctors had little or no education in nutrition and diet. In fact, until the late twentieth century, most allopathically-trained doctors didn't even recognize the role nutrition played in health. My, how quickly times change! Unfortunately, for far too many years most Americans (and doctors, for that matter) interpreted this advice of eating a balanced diet to mean eating some *good* food and some *bad* food. Again, this is more garbage. It's very reminiscent of the *"everything in moderation"* slogan fat-sick people often espouse. Most Americans think a balanced diet means a salad and a candy bar; something good and something bad, something healthy and something unhealthy.

The original intent of a *balanced* diet was a diet consisting entirely of "food," *never* doof. A balanced diet consisted of *all* good foods *in balance* to one another. It meant a balancing of basic food groups, like fruits, vegetables, and legumes with meat, dairy, and starches. It never meant to include doof like ice cream, soda, energy bars and French fries. Doof isn't a food group. Doof isn't part of a "balanced" diet. In fact, it's really the opposite of balance, isn't it?

America's Warped Perception of a "Balanced" Diet

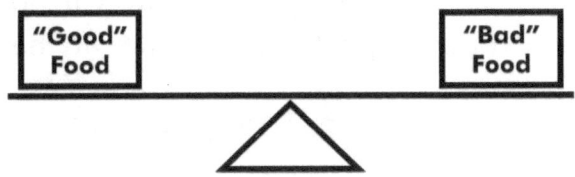

Be honest with yourself and start to eat a *healthy* diet. Stay away from the misconception of a *balanced* diet at all costs. Doing so will help keep you healthy and slim.

Principle 11: Discipline at the Store, *Not* the Frig

Discipline occurs at the grocery store, not half asleep, in front of the refrigerator at 3 a.m. People often say they don't have any discipline and can't help eating doof. They say they get up at 3 a.m. and binge in front of the refrigerator. Again, when trying to help someone, I may ask them:

"When you're lacking discipline, where does the food come from?"

"What do you mean where does it come from?" they ask, perplexed?

"I mean, from where do you get the food?"

The Honesty Diet

"From my refrigerator. Where else?"

"How did the doof get into your refrigerator?" I question further.

"I bought it at the store."

"Did you open the doof and start eating it in the store?"

"No."

"So you had the discipline not to tear open the package and start gobbling it down at the store, right?"

"Yeah. Well, I wasn't craving it when I was at the store."

"If you were craving it then, would you have opened the item in the store?"

"No. Not until after I'd paid for it."

"So you did have discipline in the store. You're not an animal," I say. "Then why did you buy it if you knew it's a bad food?"

"I don't' know. Because I *wanted* it. I guess I figured I would just eat some later."

"But you don't have 'just eat some' later. You eat the whole thing, don't you?"

"Sometimes."

"Well, your behavior suggests you don't really *want* to be healthy. You claim not to have the discipline to keep yourself from eating something bad while standing in front of your refrigerator, but then you admit you *do* have the discipline when you're at the store."

"So? What are you getting at?"

"Discipline occurs at the grocery store, not in front

of your refrigerator. You do have the discipline. We know that because you exhibit it at the grocery store. The truth is you really don't *want* to be healthy. You're perfectly content being fat-sick."

Your level of awareness at the grocery store is critical. It is important you set yourself up to win when you shop for groceries. First, I recommend you eat a little bit of real food *before* you go to the store. That way you're not starving when you go in and won't be tempted to buy doof while you shop. Second, I recommend you dress up before you shop for groceries. Seriously. I have noticed the better I feel about myself when I shop, the better food selections I tend to make. Dressing well makes me feel good about myself. So for guys, that means, shaving, and wearing some nice clothes to the grocery store. For ladies, that might mean fixing your hair and wearing something that makes you feel good about yourself. Besides, you never know, you might just meet that someone special, run into an old friend, or a prospective employer while food shopping. You wouldn't want to look like a slob, would you? I think you'll be surprised to discover the better you feel about yourself when you shop, the healthier decisions you'll tend to make for yourself. Discipline occurs at the grocery store, not in your home.

Getting the Big Picture: The Final Awareness

The final principle sums up The Honesty Diet in a single statement. It is a concept that has been obvious to me for over a decade, but one I have been unable to succinctly communicate. It was so obvious that, in retrospect, I can't believe it took me so long to find a way to articulate it effectively.

For over a decade, I have collected hundreds of articles from medical journals and health magazines reporting the results of countless numbers of studies on various kinds of foods and their subsequent health benefits. However, I have never come across any honest studies stating conclusions such as:

- French fries prevent cancer.
- Candy bars reduce heart cancer risk.
- Trans-fats lower cholesterol.
- Fast-food reduces pain.

On the other hand, I do find countless studies concluding:

- Blueberries help prevent urinary tract infections.
- Carrots help prevent colon cancer and stroke.
- Strawberries help prevent heart disease.
- Nuts help prevent gall stones and diabetes.
- Bananas help prevent anemia and strokes.
- Kale helps prevent breast cancer and lung cancer.
- Oranges help prevent cardiovascular disease.
- Avocados help prevent obesity and hypertension.
- Spinach helps prevent cataracts and birth defects.

The list seems endless. There is absolutely no shortage of these kinds of studies out there. The only problem with all of these studies is they represent an effort to

Don't Take Advice From Fat Doctors!

micromanage one's nutritional health. For example, if a woman wants to prevent cataracts, she may choose to overdose on spinach, but continue to eat fast-food on a regular basis. She then may wonder why she developed cataracts anyway. Or, a man may want to avoid heart disease by eating several oranges everyday, but he never exercises. He then wonders why he still developed heart disease. You see? You can't micro-manage nutrition. You cannot micromanage health. You must be honest. You must recognize the final principle.

The answer is so obvious it escapes most of us. And the answer couldn't possibly be any more simple. The final awareness is…

Principle 12: Food prevents disease, Doof causes disease

You see? We don't need hundreds of studies suggesting blueberries help prevent cataracts, zucchini prevents heart attacks, broccoli contains nutrients that can help fight cancer, or that apples boost your immune system. We just need to be honest and stop eating doof! Can you see the bigger picture? *Food* prevents disease. *Doof* causes disease. So, eat food. Could it possibly be any simpler? Another way of expressing this principle is:

Food causes health. Doof causes disease.

> *"If we eat wrongly, no doctor can cure us.
> If we eat rightly, no doctor is needed."*
>
> - attributed to Dr. Victor G. Rocine

Principle Summary

1. Be Honest and *Think*!
2. *Eat* More Water, Don't *Drink* More Water!
3. Don't Confuse "Full" With "Nourished"
4. Eat Food, Not Doof™
5. Your Refrigerator *Is* Your Body
6. Eat Those *In*expensive Organic Foods
7. Read Labels Carefully
8. The Fewer Ingredients the Better
9. Avoid "Everything in Moderation"
10. Eat a "Healthy," Not a "Balanced" Diet
11. Discipline at the Store, *Not* the Frig
12. Food Prevents Disease, Doof Causes Disease

~ 24 ~

DECIDE

Rather than write a closing rah-rah "you can do it" pep talk, let me just reiterate that what has been presented in this book is a *set of beliefs* that, when acted upon, can produce tremendous physical and psychological change in a person's life.

People frequently create fictitious obstacles, like finding exceptions to the awarenesses and principles I have suggested in The Honesty Diet, so they can have an excuse not to change. In fact, I have observed fat-sick people are almost always looking for the exception to everything. They are full of "Yeah, buts." For example, smoking causes lung cancer. However, most of us can think of someone who smoked all their life and never developed lung cancer. That's good news, but it is beside the point. The fact of the matter is nothing is absolute, and nothing exists in a vacuum. But people who do not *want* to grow and change often *look for the exception* because they want to try to disprove an often uncomfortable suggestion or assertion put forth by a doctor or other healthcare professional.

If one were looking for a reason *not* to change, one could *easily* find fault with *any* of the beliefs or contentions presented in this book. But doing that probably wouldn't serve one's health. The issue isn't whether or not the beliefs presented here are absolutely true and accurate under any and all conceivable circumstances. Although I personally think they are true and accurate, that doesn't mean someone else couldn't disagree with them and/or find fault with them. However, those who follow these beliefs, whether provable or not and regardless if some other "expert" can find fault with them or not, have the capacity to produce incredibly beneficial changes that can dramatically improve your life, your health, and the quality of both.

A Final Yeah, but: "It Can't Be That Easy"

"It can't be that easy" is the most common "Yeah, but" I hear. No doubt there will be people who criticize some, or all, of this book as being "too simplistic." I would ask you to consider the notion that when most people say something is "too simplistic," what they are really doing is making an excuse for not changing.

A mentor of mine once said to me, "Sometimes you have to make excuses to do things... instead of excuses to *not* do things." Most people make excuses to *not* do things. One of the ways they rationalize this is by saying a task is "too" something. However, instead of saying something that might make someone look like a wimp, like, "it's too *hard,*" a person will swing to the other end of the intellectual pendulum and say, "it's too *simplistic,*" as if this makes the "Yeah, but" any more valid. It doesn't.

Others may deem this book "too extreme." However, this "Yeah, but" is *evidence* of the current sickness of the country. I would offer that what we've been doing to ourselves, have become accustomed to, and the dire predicament we have put ourselves in, are the real signs of extremism. The way the general public is living now is extreme and is the *cause* of our plight – not the rational philosophy I am proposing! Only a nation as fat and sick as ours could possibly interpret my basic, mild, easy suggestions as "extreme."

The more you read the beliefs contained in this book, the more you repeat them to yourself and to others, and the more you accept and practice them, the more you will reprogram your brain to intuitively seek out health instead of fatness and sickness. The Honesty Diet really is – not extreme, not simplistic – but *extremely simple!* Once your brain accepts the beliefs herein as valid, it will become immeasurably easier to make better daily health decisions.

I would argue that you may have been living by another set of beliefs that has produced the body you see in the mirror today and the health you experience on a daily basis. My question to you is this: *Is your current system of beliefs honestly serving you, or not?* If the answer is no, I suggest that you consider a new set of beliefs, perhaps similar to those I have presented throughout this book.

About the Author

Dr. Sean Hannon is a chiropractic doctor who left health care practice many years ago upon finally recognizing and accepting the reality that most people do not want to be healthy. The Honesty Diet is a product of his insights and frustrations in practice and of his own struggle with a serious spine injury that left him unable to walk for over a year.

Dr. Hannon earned a bachelor's degree in the 1990s. He left a successful corporate sales career in New York City to complete his pre-medical education and doctorate at the turn of the century. During his training in South Carolina, Dr. Hannon frequently presented to the faculty and student body on the subjects of contemporary chiropractic research and personal effectiveness. He was a featured speaker at the 9th Annual Vertebral Subluxation Conference in 2001, and completed his clinical internship that same year. His more than 300 hours of post-doctoral studies have almost exclusively focused on the role micro-nutrition plays in the prevention of common degenerative diseases.

Dr. Hannon is the recipient of the B.J. Palmer Philosophy Award and is a two-time winner of the national John Starchurski Memorial Award. His first professional, peer-reviewed research paper was published in the April 2004 issue of the Journal of Vertebral Subluxation Research. This same research paper was subsequently presented by peers at conferences in Washington, DC and Australia, was featured in numerous professional trade journals, and was incorporated into the research curriculum at Life University in Marietta, Georgia.

In 2002, Dr. Hannon's work was a contributing resource to a National Institute of Health (NIH) grant proposal on genetic expression submitted by researchers at Colorado State University (CSU), and is a cited reference in the 2003 Clinical Practices Guidelines officially registered with the Library of Congress.

No longer in practice, Dr. Hannon has owned and operated for more than a decade a multi-award-winning martial arts school exclusively for adults near Denver, Colorado. His business has been featured in numerous national and international publications including *The Wall Street Journal*.

Also by Sean Hannon

Inner Bushido
Strength Without Conflict

C.I.P.A. EVVY Award Winner 2014

www.ingramcontent.com/pod-product-compliance
Lightning Source LLC
Chambersburg PA
CBHW022058120526
44592CB00033B/134